The Big Ketogenic Cookbook

the big KETOGENIC cookbook

delicious & nutritious keto diet recipes

high fat low carb cookbook for
breakfast, lunch, dinner & dessert

Recipes365

• BEFORE YOU BEGIN •

Free Bonus Guide: Top 10 Keto Diet Mistakes

We've put together a free companion guide to go with this recipe book. It features the top 10 mistakes made by people on the ketogenic diet.

If you want to avoid costly mistakes and accelerate your progress you will find a link to the guide at the back of this book. If you can't wait that long, see below now!

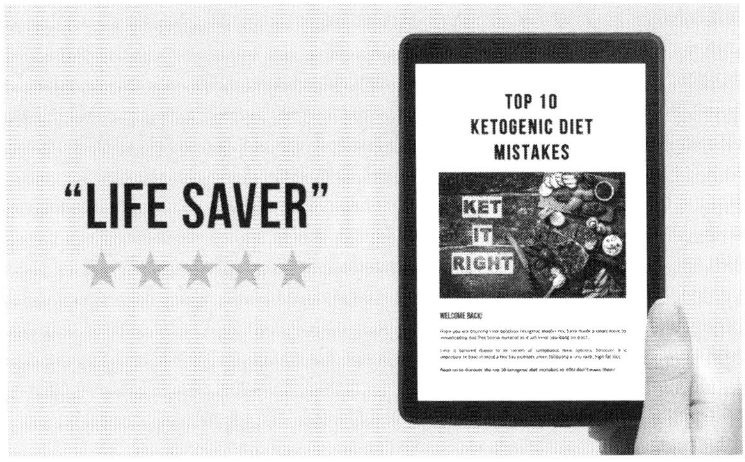

Visit http://geni.us/ketomistakes to get your copy now!

Table of Contents

Introduction

Hello there!

Welcome to a wonderful 120 ketogenic breakfasts, lunches, dinners and desserts! By now you are probably well aware of the benefits of going keto but just in case you need to refresh your memory, here's a quick top-up before we dive right into the recipes.

The Science in a Nutshell

Your body normally converts carbohydrates to glucose for energy. By limiting your intake and replacing it with fats, your body enters a state of ketosis.

Here your body produces ketones, created by a breakdown of fats in the liver. Without carbohydrates as your primary source of energy your body will turn to the ketones instead.

This effectively cranks up the fat burning furnace and puts your body in the ultimate metabolic state.

What Keto Can do for You

Keto has its origins in treating healthcare conditions such as epilepsy, type 2 diabetes, cardiovascular disease, metabolic syndrome, auto-brewery syndrome and high blood pressure but now has much wider application in weight control.

This diet, then, will take you above and beyond typical results and propel you into a new realm of total body health. If you want to look and feel the best you possibly can, all without sacrificing your love of delicious food, then this is the cookbook for you.

Things to Remember

A healthy diet is not solution to anything in and of itself; it must be applied as part of a healthy lifestyle in order to see maximum results.

Think of the ketogenic diet as the foundation of your new body. If you want to build something truly special on top of it then design your lifestyle with that goal in mind.

Cutting out junk food goes without saying, as does ditching bad habits such as smoking and drinking. Exercise, too, will take you to heights you never thought was possible.

So, as you explore these delectable dishes and embark on the keto diet, try not to neglect other areas or responsibility.

Let this be the start of something great!

The Recipes

We wanted to make it as simple as possible for you to get in the kitchen and rustle up something special, so you will find each recipe laid out in an easy to follow format.

Each begins with a short intro to the dish, followed by the serving size and list of ingredients. Remember, this diet is designed to rekindle your love of food not extinguish it with rules and regulations, so don't be afraid to experiment.

Use the ingredients as general guidelines and follow the instructions as best you can. You may not get everything perfect first time, every time but that is what makes it yours!

Keep at it for a full 30 days of eating and you will no doubt establish a few firm favorites that you can turn into your specialty dishes over time.

Each recipe ends with a breakdown of key nutritional information including number of calories and amount of fats, carbohydrates and protein.

Again, this isn't to be obsessed over. Food is something to be enjoyed, so if you are going to keep note of your intake levels then just make it a general estimate.

Why no pics? This cookbook is full of *fun* and *flavor*, and doesn't take itself too seriously. The food is entering your mouth, not a modeling contest, and we don't like to encourage unhealthy obsession about presentation. So just cook, experiment, and enjoy.

Once you start loving what you are eating mealtimes will become something to look forward to. Take this as encouragement, go forth and cook to your heart's content!

Breakfasts

Keto Cream Cheese Pancakes

SERVES 8-10

4 eggs

4 oz. cream cheese, softened

1 tbsp. sugar substitute

2 tsp. vanilla extract

4 tbsp. coconut flour

1½ tsp. baking powder

Almond milk as needed

Yes, you can have pancakes on the keto diet! You're one recipe in and probably already beginning to understand why it's so popular.

1. Combine the eggs, cream cheese, sugar substitute, and vanilla with a blender or mixer.

2. Add the coconut flour and baking powder. Combine well. If the batter thickens after a few minutes, add a little almond milk to thin it.

3. Heat the electric griddle to 325°F. Pour the batter in 5-inch circles.

4. Wait for the surface to bubble, and then flip. Cook for 2-4 minutes longer, or until browned.

5. Serve with the toppings of your choice, or use for sandwiches.

NUTRITIONAL INFO PER SERVING

Calories: 100

Fat: 8g

Net Carbs: 3.5g

Protein: 5g

Delicious Coconut Flour Waffles

SERVES 5

4 tbsp. coconut flour

5 eggs, separated by white and yolk

1 tsp. baking powder

4-5 tbsp. granulated stevia or your own sweetener

3 tbsp. whole milk

1 tsp. vanilla

4½ oz. butter, melted

Super hungry and in a rush? This recipe takes only few minutes! Accept the challenge to eat just one. It works well with any topping, and even the kids will love it!

1. Whisk the egg whites in a bowl until they form stiff peaks.

2. In another bowl, mix the egg yolk with the coconut flour, the stevia or sweetener, and the baking powder.

3. Add the melted butter. Do so slowly, mixing until the batter is smooth.

4. Add the milk and the vanilla.

5. Combine the mixture of the first bowl with the second one, folding it in to keep the fluffiness of the batter.

6. When the waffle maker is warmed up, pour in some waffle mixture. When it is golden brown, it's finished. Repeat until all the batter is used.

NUTRITIONAL INFO PER SERVING

Calories: 277

Fat: 22g

Net Carbs: 4.3g

Protein: 8g

Healthy Vegetable Breakfast Hash

SERVES 1

1 medium zucchini

¼ cup white onion

2 oz. bacon

1 tbsp. coconut oil

Fresh parsley, chopped

1 large egg

Salt to taste

Bacon and veggies will be sure to brighten your morning! Replace the eggs with avocado for an egg-free alternative.

1. Slice the bacon, and peel and dice the onion and zucchini.

2. Sauté the onion over medium heat and add the bacon. Stir and cook until slightly browned.

3. Add the zucchini to the pan, and cook for 10-15 minutes.

4. When done, place the hash on a plate and add the chopped parsley.

5. Top with a fried egg or, for an egg-free version, avocado.

NUTRITIONAL INFO PER SERVING

Calories: 427

Fat: 35g

Net Carbs: 7g

Protein: 17g

Yummy Avocado and Salmon Breakfast Boats

Serves 1

1 avocado

1 oz. fresh goat cheese

2 oz. smoked salmon

2 tbsp. lemon juice

2 tbsp. of organic extra virgin olive oil

A dash of sea salt

Salmon and avocado are both good and healthy fat sources for your keto diet. Here, they combine for an exquisite breakfast option.

1. Cut the avocado in half, removing the stone.

2. Mix the rest of the ingredients – the salmon, goat cheese, oil, lemon juice, and salt - in a food processor until they have a creamy consistency, and place the mixture inside the avocado.

3. Enjoy!

Nutritional Info per Serving

Calories: 520

Fat: 45g

Net Carbs: 5g

Protein: 20g

Sausage Casserole with Vegetables

SERVES 6

2 cups zucchini, diced

¼ cup onion, diced

1 lb. pork sausage

2 cups cabbage, shredded

3 eggs

2 tbsp. mustard

½ cup mayonnaise

1½ cups cheddar cheese, shredded

1 tbsp. dried ground sage

Cayenne pepper

The whole family will enjoy this awesome breakfast casserole. It takes less than an hour to make and keeps you satisfied all morning long, so perhaps one for a lazy Sunday.

1. Preheat the oven to 375°F. Grease a casserole dish and set it aside.

3. In a large skillet on a medium heat, cook the sausage and the veggies until tender.

4. Place the mixture into the casserole dish.

5. In a separate bowl, mix the eggs, mustard, mayonnaise, sage, and pepper until combined well.

6. Add the grated cheese to the egg mixture and stir for 1 minute.

7. Pour the mix over the sausage and vegetables in the casserole dish, and top with the cheese.

8. Bake the casserole for 30 minutes, or remove it when it is bubbling around the edges and the cheese on the top is melted.

NUTRITIONAL INFO PER SERVING

Calories: 480

Fat: 42g

Net Carbs: 5g

Protein: 20g

Keto Lemon Muffins with Poppy Seeds

Serves 12

¾ cup almond flour

⅓ cup Erythritol

¼ cup Flaxseed meal

1 tbsp. baking powder

2 tbsp. poppy seeds

¼ cup Butter, melted

3 eggs

¼ cup Heavy cream

3 tbsp. lemon juice

Lemon zest of 2 lemons

1 tbsp. vanilla

20 drops liquid sweetener

There's nothing better than the taste of lemon and poppy seed muffins to refresh you in the morning. Fast to make and easy to store, they can be part of your breakfast (or late morning snacks) throughout the week. Plus, they're low-carb!

1. Preheat the oven to 345°F.

2. Meanwhile, mix in a bowl the flaxseed meal, almond flour, erythritol and poppy seeds.

3. Add melted butter, and mix in the eggs and heavy cream until it reaches a smooth consistency. Add the rest of the ingredients and mix.

4. Place the batter into the muffin pan (divided into 12) and bake them for 18-20 minutes.

5. Remove from the oven and cool for approximately 10 minutes.

Nutritional Info per Serving

Calories: 130

Fat: 11.5g

Net Carbs: 1.7g

Protein: 4g

Breakfast Tacos

SERVES 3

1 cup mozzarella cheese, shredded

6 eggs

2 tbsp. butter

3 strips of bacon

1 oz. cheddar cheese, shredded

½ an avocado

Salt and pepper

A grab-and-go breakfast! You will be delighted by the crunchy cheese taco shell and the huge variety of fillings you can use with it.

1. Cook the bacon on a baking sheet covered with aluminum foil at 375°F, until crispy (12-15 minutes).

2. Meanwhile, use a third of the mozzarella to cover the bottom of a nonstick pan. Heat for 2-3 minutes on medium heat, or until the edges begin to brown.

3. With a pair of tongs, remove the mozzarella from the pan (it will now be a taco shell). Repeat with the remaining cheese.

4. Scramble the eggs in the butter. Stir frequently, and add pepper and salt to taste.

5. Fill the shells with the eggs, avocado and bacon. Sprinkle cheddar cheese on the top. Add hot sauce or cilantro (optional).

NUTRITIONAL INFO PER SERVING

Calories: 440

Fat: 36g

Net Carbs: 4g

Protein: 26g

Cheddar and Bacon Omelets with Chives

Serves 1

2 slices of bacon

2 tbsp. bacon grease

2 eggs

2 stalks of chives

1 oz. cheddar cheese

Salt and pepper

Chives always give a unique flavor to your food – and it's even better with cheddar and bacon! This recipe is super easy, and super delicious.

1. Place the bacon fat in a pre-heated pan on a medium-low heat, and let it melt. Add the eggs, chives, salt and pepper. Stir lightly.

2. Add the bacon once the edges are set. Cook for 20-30 seconds more.

3. Add cheese to the omelet and fold in half. Flip over and warm through on the other side.

Nutritional Info per Serving

Calories: 460

Fat: 40g

Net Carbs: 2g

Protein: 25g

Pumpkin Bread

SERVES 10

1½ cups almond flour

3 egg whites

¼ cup granulated sugar

½ cup coconut milk

¼ cup psyllium husk powder

1½ tsp. pumpkin pie spice

2 tsp. baking powder

½ tsp. salt

If you're a pumpkin lover and missing all the Halloween pumpkin treats, you're going to love this loaf. Each serving acts like a delicious little protein bar.

1. In a bowl, sift all the dry ingredients. Place a container with 1 cup of water into a preheated oven (350°F).

2. Add the pumpkin and coconut milk to the dry ingredients, and mix.

3. Whisk the egg whites, and add them into the dough, folding carefully.

4. Place the dough into a greased loaf pan, and cook the bread for 75 minutes.

NUTRITIONAL INFO PER SERVING

Calories: 120

Fat: 9g

Net Carbs: 3g

Protein: 5g

Salted Caramel Cereal with Pork Rinds

Serves 1

1 oz. pork rinds

2 tbsp. butter

1 cup vanilla coconut milk

2 tbsp. heavy cream

¼ tbsp. ground cinnamon

1 tbsp. erythritol

This crunch, salty-sweet combination will knock your socks off in the morning, which is inconvenient if you've only just put them on. Oh well.

1. In a pan on a medium heat, add the butter and stir until browned.

2. Remove and add the heavy cream and erythritol. Mix well and return to the heat. Continue heating, stirring constantly until the desired caramel color is achieved.

3. Add the pork rinds and mix them in, being careful to coat evenly.

4. Place them into a container and put in the fridge for 20-45 minutes to cool them down.

Nutritional Info per Serving

Calories: 510

Fat: 50g

Net Carbs: 2.7g

Protein: 15g

Red Chocolate Doughnuts

Serves 9

For the donut:

¼ cup Erythritol

½ cup coconut flour

2 tbsp. cocoa powder

¼ cup coconut oil

½ cup coconut milk

½ tbsp. vanilla extract

¼ tsp. salt

¼ tsp. baking soda

4 eggs

¼ tsp. apple cider vinegar

¼ tsp. liquid stevia

1 tsp. red food coloring

For the icing:

¼ cup powdered erythritol

4 oz. cream cheese

4 tbsp. butter

2 tbsp. heavy cream

½ tsp. vanilla extract

1 tsp. red food coloring

Chocolate, vanilla and coconut come together to make red velvet like you've never tasted before – and in a way that you won't feel too guilty for eating one...or two.

1. Sift the coconut flour, cocoa powder, salt and baking soda, and mix.

2. Mix the eggs, erythritol, vanilla, coconut oil, coconut milk and red food coloring. Add them into the dry ingredients and mix again.

3. Divide the batter between the molds in the donut tray. Bake in a preheated oven at 335°F for 16-18 minutes.

4. Remove the donuts from the trays and cool for 10 minutes.

5. In a pan, heat the coconut oil to its smoking point and fry the donuts on both sides. Drain them in a paper towel.

6. Combine the butter, cream cheese, heavy cream, vanilla and powdered erythritol, beating until it has a fluffy consistency. Add the food coloring, mix again, and frost the donuts.

Nutritional Info per Serving

Calories: 150
Fat: 15g
Net Carbs: 2g
Protein: 2g

Cheddar Scrambled Eggs with Spinach

SERVES 1

4 cup fresh spinach

4 eggs

½ cup cheddar cheese

1 tbsp. heavy cream

1 tbsp. olive oil

Salt and pepper

This breakfast provides you all the nutrients needed to start off a wonderful day. Green never tasted so good!

1. In a bowl, mix together the eggs, heavy cream, salt and pepper.
2. Heat a large pan, and add the olive oil and spinach when the oil is heated.
3. Stir the spinach, and add the salt and pepper.
4. Once the spinach is fairly wilted, add the egg mixture and turn to medium heat.
5. When the eggs are set, add the cheese and stir slowly until it melts.

NUTRITIONAL INFO PER SERVING

Calories: 700

Fat: 58g

Net Carbs: 5g

Protein: 43g

Brownie Muffins for Ketoheads

Serves 6

1 cup golden flaxseed meal

1 tbsp. cinnamon

¼ cup cocoa powder

½ tsp. salt

½ tsp. baking powder

1 egg

2 tbsp. coconut oil

¼ cup sugar-free caramel syrup

½ cup pumpkin purée

1 tbsp. vanilla extract

1 tbsp. apple cider vinegar

¼ cup slivered almonds

These muffins look like chocolate but they aren't! And why is that a good thing? Because you can eat them shamelessly. Made with wholesome ingredients, they are perfect for an everyday breakfast.

1. Preheat oven to 350°F.

2. Place all the ingredients except the almonds into a large mixing bowl, and combine well.

3. In a lined muffin pan, fill each space, dividing the batter into 6 parts.

4. Sprinkle the almonds on top.

5. Bake for around 15 minutes.

Nutritional Info per Serving

Calories: 185

Fat: 13.5g

Net Carbs: 3.5g

Protein: 7.4g

Sausage and Bacon Bite Sized Breakfasts

SERVES 1

6 slices bacon

6 oz. breakfast sausage

1 tbsp. butter

6 eggs

½ tbsp. olive oil

¾ stalk celery

2 stalks leek

⅕ onion

Salt and pepper

If you like sausages, and you like bacon, and you also like convenience... then you'll love these rich bite-sized breakfast pieces!

1. In a food processor, mix the bacon and sausage together. Place the mixture into a cupcake tray, filling each cup to the top, and making a slight indent in the top of each. Bake for 15 minutes at 375°F.

2. Dice the leeks and celery, and add them to the buttered pan. Season with salt and pepper. Sauté until the celery and leeks are fairly tender. Remove the mixture from the pan and re-use the butter to fry the eggs.

3. Take the sausage bites from oven. Drain any excess oil with a paper towel, and bake again for 10 minutes.

4. Remove the baskets and fill them with the onion-leek mixture. Set the fried egg on top and serve.

NUTRITIONAL INFO PER SERVING

Calories: 239

Fat: 20g

Net Carbs: 2g

Protein: 15g

Italian Sausage and Egg Scramble

SERVES 1

1 cup red bell pepper, chopped

1 cup onion, chopped

4 eggs

3 spicy Italian chicken sausages

¼ cup mozzarella cheese, shredded

1 tsp. cayenne pepper powder

Salt

When you have no idea what to cook for a nice breakfast, check out this recipe. Not only is it super easy, but it's super delicious – we're sure you will love it!

1. Place the chopped red bell peppers and onion into a skillet. Sauté until the onion starts to turn transparent, and then add the chicken sausage (chopped into small pieces).

2. Sauté just long enough to heat the sausage.

3. Add the eggs and mozzarella cheese, and mix with a spatula.

4. Scramble for a further 3-4 minutes, or until the mixture has finished cooking.

5. Add the cayenne pepper and salt to taste.

NUTRITIONAL INFO PER SERVING

Calories: 750

Fat: 40g

Net Carbs: 17g

Protein: 75g

Versatile Oopsie Rolls

SERVES 6

Cooking spray

6 oz. cream cheese, cold and cubed

6 eggs

¼ tsp. cream of tartar

¼ tsp. salt

Popular among the keto community, these rolls are very versatile. Add your own personal touch and let them be the star of your breakfast sandwich, breakfast pizza, and more!

1. Separate the egg whites and yolks. Whisk the whites with an electric hand mixer until they are foamy.

2. Add cream of tartar, and keep mixing until they start to form stiff peaks.

3. In another bowl, mix the egg yolks with cream cheese until smooth, and then carefully fold in the white egg mixture.

4. Place the batter on a cookie sheet with parchment paper.

5. Bake for about 30-40 minutes and cool.

NUTRITIONAL INFO PER SERVING

Calories: 45

Fat: 4g

Net Carbs: 0g

Protein: 2.5g

Keto Crepes with Blueberries

SERVES 6

For the Crepe Batter:

2 oz. cream cheese

2 eggs

10 drops liquid stevia

¼ tsp. cinnamon

¼ tsp. baking soda

⅛ tsp. salt

For the Filling:

4 oz. cream cheese

½ tsp. vanilla extract

2 tsp. powdered erythritol

½ cup blueberries

Here's one to help you out when you've got to make a quick breakfast. Though crepes can be eaten with anything, try out this blueberry filling for a breakfast you'll want to repeat!

1. In a bowl, mix the cream cheese and eggs with an electric hand mixer until smooth.

2. Add the stevia, cinnamon, baking soda and salt, and mix.

3. Add butter or coconut oil in a nonstick pan, and heat over medium. Pour in some batter – to make a very thin layer - and cook for 3 minutes. Flip the crepe, cook for a further minute, and remove.

4. Make the filling: combine the cream cheese, vanilla extract and powdered erythritol, and stir with the electric mixer until creamy.

5. Add the filling, cinnamon and blueberries to your crepes and either fold or roll them up.

NUTRITIONAL INFO PER SERVING

Calories: 400

Fat: 35g

Net Carbs: 6g

Protein: 15g

Keto Cheddar and Sage Waffle

Serves 12

1⅓ cups coconut flour

3 tbsp. baking powder

1 tsp. ground sage, dried

½ tsp. salt

¼ tsp. garlic powder

2 cups canned coconut milk

½ cup water

2 eggs

3 tbsp. coconut oil, melted

1 cup cheddar cheese, shredded

Waffles are good with syrup, and even better savory! Try this option out as a sandwich, or with a cheese sauce, guacamole, or gravy.

1. Mix the flour, baking powder and seasonings together in a bowl.

2. Add the coconut milk, water and coconut oil and beat them until they form a stiff batter.

3. Combine with the cheese.

4. Grease and heat the waffle iron, and pour onto each iron section ⅓ cup of the batter.

5. Close the iron until the waffles are browned.

Nutritional Info per Serving

Calories: 214

Fat: 17.2g

Net Carbs: 3.8g

Protein: 6.5g

Keto Casserole for Breakfast

Serves 8

¼ cup flaxseed meal

1 cup almond flour

10 eggs

1 lb. breakfast sausage

4 oz. cheese

6 tbsp. light maple syrup

4 tbsp. butter

½ tsp. onion powder

½ tsp. garlic powder

¼ tsp. sage

Salt and pepper

Casseroles are famous for being easy – this one is no exception.

1. In a pan on medium heat, add the breakfast sausage, stirring frequently, until browned.

2. In a bowl, mix the flaxseed, almond flour, onion powder, garlic powder and sage together.

3. Add the eggs and cheese to the bowl, and mix.

4. Add this mixture to the sausage.

5. Line a casserole dish with parchment paper, and pour in the casserole mix. Drizzle the 2 tbsp. of syrup on top.

6. Bake at 350°F for about 45-55 minutes and cool.

Nutritional Info per Serving

Calories: 480

Fat: 41.2g

Net Carbs: 3g

Protein: 22.7g

Breakfast Burgers

SERVES 2

4 oz. sausage

2 oz. pepper jack cheese

4 slices bacon

2 eggs

1 tbsp. butter

1 tbsp. peanut butter powder

Salt and pepper

For those who like a heavy breakfast, this is a great option. Combining sweet and savory, it's a very unique option that you're sure to enjoy.

1. Bake the bacon on a cooking sheet at 400°F for 20-25 minutes.

2. Combine the butter and peanut butter powder in a small bowl.

3. Form 2 patties from the sausage, and cook them until well done.

4. Add cheese, and cover with a lid so that it melts. Remove from the pan.

5. Cook the egg and set atop the burger along with the peanut butter mix and bacon slices.

NUTRITIONAL INFO PER SERVING

Calories: 652

Fat: 55g

Net Carbs: 3g

Protein: 30g

Peanut Butter Muffins with Chocolate Chips

SERVES 2

½ cup erythritol

1 cup almond flour

1 tbsp. baking powder

⅓ cup almond milk

⅓ cup peanut butter

2 eggs

½ cup sugar-free chocolate chips

Salt

These muffins are an easy grab-and-go breakfast. A rich peanut butter flavor – and a sugar-free one, at that – is sure to get rid of your cravings.

1. Mix the erythritol, almond flour, and baking powder in a bowl and whisk.

2. Add the peanut butter and almond milk, and stir.

3. Add in the first egg and combine well. Add the second and combine well.

3. Fold in the chocolate chips.

4. Place the muffins in a muffin tin (of 6 cups) and bake them on 350°F for 15 minutes and cool.

NUTRITIONAL INFO PER SERVING

Calories: 527

Fat: 40g

Net Carbs: 4.3g

Protein: 14g

Keto Green Smoothie

Serves 1

1½ cups almond milk

1 oz. spinach

⅓ cup cucumber, diced

⅓ cup celery, diced

½ cup avocado, diced

1 tbsp. coconut oil

Liquid stevia

¼ cup protein powder

This awesome smoothie does not have any fruit in it! It takes just a couple of minutes to make, and will give you the nutrients you need to have an energetic morning.

1. Blend the almond milk and spinach in a blender.

2. Make room for the rest of the ingredients, and blend again until a smooth consistency is achieved.

Nutritional Info per Serving

Calories: 370

Fat: 24g

Net Carbs: 5g

Protein: 27g

Keto Oatmeal

SERVES 2

¼ cup shredded coconut, unsweetened

⅓ cup almonds, flaked

¼ cup chia seeds

⅓ cup flaked coconut, unsweetened

1 tsp. unsweetened vanilla extract

1 cup hot water

½ cup coconut milk

2 tbsp. erythritol

6-8 drops stevia extract

A whole, healthy breakfast. You won't want to miss this delicious way to treat your body well. Chia seeds are great source of healthy fats and make a lovely finishing touch.

1. In a bowl, place the flaked and shredded coconut, almonds and chia seeds, setting aside a little bit of flaked coconut and almond.

2. Add the coconut milk, vanilla extract, stevia and combine. Add hot water and let sit for 10-15 minutes.

3. Sprinkle with flaked coconuts and almonds and top with berries (optional).

NUTRITIONAL INFO PER SERVING

Calories: 360

Fat: 30 g

Net Carbs: 5 g

Protein: 9.5 g

Carrot Muffins

Serves 9

For the Cheesecake Layer:

¾ cup cream cheese

1 egg yolk

2 tbsp. erythritol

1 tsp. unsweetened vanilla extract

For the Rest:

½ cup almond flour

2 tbsp. coconut flour

1 tbsp. ground chia seeds

¼ cup Erythritol

2 tsp. gluten-free baking powder

1 tsp. each cinnamon, vanilla powder and ground ginger

⅛ tsp. each ground allspice and nutmeg

½ cup chopped pecans

5 egg whites

⅓ cup virgin coconut oil, melted

¾ cup carrots, grated

20 drops liquid stevia

Melted coconut oil for greasing

Salt

A perfect keto treat for the fall. The little cheesecake layer is simply out of this world!

1. Make the cheesecake layer by mixing together the cream cheese, egg yolk, erythritol and vanilla powder.

2. In a separate bowl, combine well all dry ingredients (except the pecans).

3. In a large bowl, place the 4 egg yolks and the egg white left over from the cheesecake layer in a bowl, along with the melted coconut oil and stevia. Mix well, then add the dry mixture slowly while mixing well.

4. In another bowl, beat 4 egg whites until stiff peaks form.

5. Gently mix with the batter ¼ of the egg whites. Then, carefully fold in the rest with a spatula. Add the carrot and pecans, trying to keep the batter as airy as possible.

6. Line a muffin tin with 9 muffin paper cups and spoon in the batter. Top each of them with a heaping tbsp. of the cheesecake mixture. Bake for 30-35 minutes to 320°F. Remove and cool.

Nutritional Info per Serving

Calories: 270

Fat: 26g

Net Carbs: 3.7g

Protein: 7g

Savory Delicious Bacon Muffins

Serves 16

5 eggs

5 bacon slices

2 tbsp. butter

½ cups almond flour

¼ cup flaxseed meal

1½ tbsp. psyllium husk powder

2 avocados

4.5 oz. Colby-Jack cheese

3 spring onions

1 tsp. garlic

1 tsp. cilantro

1 tsp. dried chives

¼ tsp. red chili flakes

1 ½ cups coconut milk

1 ½ tbsp. lemon juice

1 tsp. baking powder

Salt and pepper

This breakfast is totally original. The avocado gives it a creamy consistency, the bacon gives it a salty punch...yeah, you should stop reading this and just get to it!

1. In a bowl, combine the eggs, flax, almond flour, psyllium, spices, lemon juice, and coconut milk.

2. In a heated pan, melt the butter and cook the bacon until browned and crispy. Remove, let cool slightly and chop into small pieces.

3. Add the bacon, avocado and the rest of the ingredients, including the bacon fat, to the batter. Combine well.

3. Divide the batter into 12 greased cupcake molds; bake them at 350°F for 20-25 minutes. Remove and cook the 4 remaining muffins.

Nutritional Info per Serving

Calories: 165

Fat: 14g

Net Carbs: 1.5g

Protein: 6g

Quick Keto Scramble

SERVES 1

3 eggs, whisked

4 baby bella mushrooms

¼ cup red bell peppers

½ cup spinach

2 slices deli ham

1 tbsp. coconut oil

Salt and pepper

A simple recipe for your breakfast—but don't let the easy preparation trick you! The mushroom and ham bring this beauty to life.

1. Mince the vegetables and the ham.
2. Brown them in a frying pan with melted butter.
3. Add the eggs and seasonings, and scramble the eggs until cooked through.

NUTRITIONAL INFO PER SERVING

Calories: 350

Fat: 30g

Net Carbs: 5g

Protein: 20g

Keto Banana Pancake

SERVES 4

2 eggs

1 banana

2 tbsp. cashew nuts, ground

¼ tsp. cinnamon

¼ tsp. ground cloves

1 tbsp. extra virgin coconut oil

For the Topping:

3 tbsp. coconut cream

¼ tsp. cinnamon

This one's for the whole family. It's just as delicious in the morning as it is post-workout.

1. Whisk the eggs in a small bowl.

2. In another bowl, mash the bananas with cinnamon, ground cashew nuts and ground cloves. Add the eggs to the mixture and combine well.

3. Grease a pan, heat, and make the pancakes by pouring enough batter to make a hand-size pancake. Flip when the edges are browned and the top begins to bubble.

4. When cooked, remove and top with the coconut cream and cinnamon.

NUTRITIONAL INFO PER SERVING

Calories: 585

Fat: 45g

Net Carbs: 27g

Protein: 20g

Keto French Toast

Serves 2 loaves

14 eggs, separated

1 cup whey protein

4 oz. cream cheese, softened

1 cup unsweetened almond milk

1 tsp. vanilla

1 tsp. cinnamon

½ cup butter

½ cup Granulated sweetener of your choice

The Keto diet doesn't mean you can't indulge yourself once in a while. This is your chance to do just that, right here.

1. Make the bread by mixing 12 egg whites for about 10 minutes, or until stiff peaks form. Add whey protein stirring gently, and fold in the cream cheese.

2. Grease two bread pans and pour the batter in them. Bake for about 40-45 minutes at 325°F. Remove and let them cool. Slice them to desired thickness after they have cooled completely.

3. Combine 2 eggs in a bowl, ½ cup unsweetened almond milk, vanilla and cinnamon. Dip the bread slices in the mixture.

4. Place the bread onto a skillet and grill until lightly browned on both sides. Repeat with the rest.

5. Make the sauce: place the butter in a saucepan in high heat. When it comes to a boil, and begins to brown, add the sweetener and the other ½ cup almond milk to the pan. Stir quickly to combine, then let cool in the pan for a couple minutes before pouring into a recipient. Top the toast with it.

Nutritional Info per Serving

Calories: 125
Fat: 15g
Net Carbs: 0.7g
Protein: 6.5g

Little Red Chocolate Cakes

Serves 1

1 tbsp. coconut flour

⅓ cup almond flour

1 tbsp. beetroot powder

1 tbsp. unsweetened cocoa powder

¼ tsp. baking soda

3 tbsp. erythritol

¼ tsp. vanilla powder

¼ cup sour cream

2 eggs

2 tbsp. extra virgin coconut oil

For the Frosting:

2 tbsp. butter, room temperature

¼ cup cream cheese

1 tbsp. powdered erythritol

¼ tsp. vanilla powder

Mug cakes are oh-so-popular, and super simple. Try this delicious little number today.

Directions

1. In a bowl, mix the almond flour, coconut flour, cacao powder, beetroot powder, baking soda, erythritol and vanilla powder.

2. Add the eggs, melted coconut oil and sour cream, and combine well.

3. Place the mixture into two mugs. Microwave each of them on high for 70-90 seconds.

4. Meanwhile, prepare the frosting by mixing the butter, erythritol, cream cheese and vanilla.

5. Frost the finished mug cakes and enjoy.

Nutritional Info per Serving

Calories: 560

Fat: 55g

Net Carbs: 8g

Protein: 15g

California Style Omelet

Serves 1

2 eggs

2 bacon slices, cooked and chopped

1 oz. deli cut chicken

¼ avocado

1 tomato

1 tbsp. mayonnaise

1 tbsp. mustard

Fresh ingredients take this omelet to the next level, and with eggs, bacon and chicken included it's a protein powerhouse.

1. Beat the eggs and pour into a hot pan. Begin to scramble and season.

2. When eggs are halfway cooked, add the chicken, bacon, sliced avocado, and tomato.

3. Combine the mayo and mustard as well and drizzle inside.

4. Fold the omelet. Cook for 5 minutes or until heated through.

Nutritional Info per Serving

Calories: 417

Fat: 35g

Net Carbs: 5g

Protein: 27g

Lunches

Keto Flat Bread

SERVES 8

For the Crust:

2 cups half-and-half grated mozzarella cheese

2 tbsp. cream cheese

¾ cup almond flour

½ tsp. sea salt

⅛ tsp. dried thyme

For the Topping:

1 cup grated Mexican cheese

½ red onion, small and sliced

4 oz. low carbohydrate sliced ham, cut

¼ medium apple, unpeeled and sliced

⅛ tsp. thyme, dried

Salt and pepper

A classic recipe that will become part of your go-to lunches. This easy recipe has apples, ham and onions – a delicious pizza style combination that you *need* to try!

1. Fill a saucepan with a little water and bring to the boil, then turn the heat to low. Place the saucepan inside a metal mixing bowl to form a double boiler, and add the mozzarella cheese, cream cheese, almond flour, thyme and salt. Stir with a spatula.
2. Cook until the cheese melts, and mix the ingredients into a dough. Pour some onto a 12-inch pizza tray covered with parchment paper. Roll the dough into a ball and place onto the center of the parchment paper. Pat into a disc shape to cover the pan.
3. Place the dough and the parchment paper on the pizza pan, poking holes throughout the dough with a fork, and bake for 6-8 minutes at 425°F. Remove.
4. Spread the toppings over the flatbread, along with the cheese, onion, apple and the ham. Cover with more cheese. Season with thyme, salt and pepper.
5. Bake again at 350°F for 5-7 minutes. Remove once the cheese begins to brown. Let cool before slicing.

NUTRITIONAL INFO PER SERVING

Calories: 257
Fat: 22g
Net Carbs: 5g
Protein: 18g

Zucchini Boats

SERVES 1

2 large zucchini

2 tbsp. butter

3 oz. shredded cheddar cheese

1 cup broccoli

6 oz. shredded rotisserie chicken

1 stalk green onion

2 tbsp. sour cream

Salt and pepper

This stuffed zucchini is an amazing option for a fast and tasty lunch packed with protein.

1. Cut the zucchini in half lengthwise, scooping out the core until you are left with a boat shape.

2. Into each zucchini pour a little melted butter, season and place into the oven at 400°F, baking for about 18 minutes.

3. In a bowl, combine the chicken, broccoli and sour cream.

4. Place the chicken mixture inside the hollowed zucchinis.

5. Top with cheddar cheese and bake for an additional 10-15 minutes.

NUTRITIONAL INFO PER SERVING

Calories: 480

Fat: 35g

Net Carbs: 5g

Protein: 28g

Keto Stromboli

Serves 4

1¼ cup shredded mozzarella cheese

4 tbsp. almond flour

3 tbsp. coconut flour

1 egg

1 tsp. Italian seasoning

4 oz. ham

4 oz. cheddar cheese

Salt and pepper

Stromboli is a traditional Italian recipe that resembles folded pizza. This keto ham and cheese version is sure to delight.

1. Melt the mozzarella cheese in the microwave for about 1 minute, stirring occasionally so as not to burn it.

2. In a separate bowl, mix almond flour, coconut flour, salt, and pepper and add the melted mozzarella cheese. Mix well. Then, after letting it cool down a bit, add the eggs and combine again.

3. Place the mixture on parchment paper, laying a second layer on top. Using your hands or rolling pin, flatten it out into a rectangle.

4. Remove the top layer of paper and with a knife cut diagonal lines toward the middle of the dough. They should be cut ⅓ of the way in on one side. Then, cut diagonal lines on the other side too.

5. On the top of the dough, alternate slices of ham and cheese. Then, fold one side over, and then the other, to cover the filling.

6. Place on a baking sheet and bake at 400°F for 15-20 minutes.

Nutritional Info per Serving

Calories: 305

Fat: 22g

Net Carbs: 5g

Protein: 25g

Keto Chicken Sandwich

SERVES 2

For the Bread:

3 eggs

3 oz. cream cheese

⅛ tsp. cream of tartar

Salt

Garlic powder

For the Filling:

1 tbsp. mayonnaise

1 tsp. sriracha

2 slices bacon

3 oz. chicken

2 slices pepper jack cheese

2 grape tomatoes

¼ avocado

Make plain keto cloud bread into a sumptuous chicken sandwich. Bacon and avocado make it even more heavenly.

1. Separate the eggs in different bowls. In the egg whites add cream tartar, salt and beat until stiff peaks form.

2. In another bowl, beat the egg yolks with cream cheese. Incorporate the mixture into the egg white mixture and combine carefully.

3. Place the batter on a parchment paper and form little square shapes that look like bread slices. Sparkle garlic powder on top and bake at 300°F for 25 minutes.

4. While the bread is baking, cook the chicken and bacon in a frying pan, seasoning to taste.

5. When the bread is done, remove from oven and let cool for 10-15 minutes. Then, make the sandwich with the cooked chicken and bacon, adding the mayo, sriracha, tomatoes, cheese and mashed avocado to taste.

NUTRITIONAL INFO PER SERVING

Calories: 360

Fat: 28g

Net Carbs: 3g

Protein: 22g

Tuna Bites with Avocado

Serves 8

10 oz. drained canned tuna

¼ cup mayo

1 avocado

¼ cup parmesan cheese

⅓ cup almond flour

½ tsp. garlic powder

¼ tsp. onion powder

½ cup coconut oil

Salt and pepper

These unique tuna bites can be served alongside a fresh salad. The avocado packs a fantastic Omega 3 fat punch!

1. In a bowl mix all the ingredients (except coconut oil). Form little balls and cover with almond flour.

2. Fry them in a pan medium heat with melted coconut oil (it has to be hot) until they seem browned on all sides.

Nutritional Info per Serving

Calories: 137

Fat: 12g

Net Carbs: 10g

Protein: 6g

Keto Green Salad

Serves 1

2 oz. mixed greens

3 tbsp. roasted pine nuts

2 tbsp. raspberry vinaigrette

2 tbsp. parmesan, shaved

2 slices bacon

Salt and pepper

Who said green salad has to be dull? These ingredients and the heavenly dressing will make your day.

1. Cook the bacon in a pan until crunchy and well browned. Break up into pieces, and add to the rest of the ingredients in a bowl.

2. Dress the salad with the raspberry vinaigrette.

Nutritional Info per Serving

Calories: 480

Fat: 37g

Net Carbs: 4g

Protein: 17g

Original Keto Stuffed Hot Dogs

SERVES 6

6 hot dogs

12 slices bacon

2 oz. cheddar

½ tsp. cheese garlic powder

½ tsp. onion powder

Salt and pepper

Have just 10 minutes for lunch? No worries, this original recipe is here to help you out!

1. Make a little slit in each hot dog, and stuff them with slices of cheese. Wrap each hot dog with 2 slices of overlapping bacon, and secure with toothpicks.

2. On top of a wire rack (with a cookie sheet below), place the hotdogs. Season them and bake at 400°F for 20-25 minutes approx.

NUTRITIONAL INFO PER SERVING

Calories: 385

Fat: 34g

Net Carbs: 0.5g

Protein: 17g

Easy Egg Soup

Serves 1

1½ cups chicken broth

½ cube of chicken bouillon

1 tbsp. bacon fat

2 eggs

1 tsp. chili garlic paste

5 minutes and 5 ingredients can make magic stuff—like this yummy egg soup.

1. In a pan on the stove on a medium-high heat, add the chicken broth, bouillon cube and bacon fat. Bring into boil and incorporate chili garlic paste and mix.

2. Whisk the eggs and add them to the chicken while stirring, then let sit for a few minutes.

Nutritional Info Per Serving

Calories: 280

Fat: 25g

Net Carbs: 2.7g

Protein: 13g

Original Nasi Lemak

Serves 2

For the Chicken & Egg:

2 chicken thighs, boneless

½ tsp. curry powder

¼ tsp. turmeric powder

½ tsp. lime juice

½ tbsp. coconut oil

1 egg

A pinch of salt

For the Nasi Lemak:

3 tbsp. coconut milk

3 slices ginger

½ small shallot

1 cup riced cauliflower

4 slices cucumber

Salt

A food with Indonesian origin, this dish will crown your lunch. It may seem complicated, but it's not too hard; and it will impress, so invite a friend to join you!

1. Rice the cauliflower and strain the water.

2. Prepare the curry powder, turmeric powder, lemon juice and salt, and marinate the chicken thighs for an hour or two in the fridge. Remove and fry.

3. Boil the coconut milk, ginger and shallot in a saucepan. When it bubbles, incorporate the cauliflower rice and mix.

4. Serve with the marinated fried chicken and fried egg.

Nutritional Info per Serving

Calories: 502

Fat: 40g

Net Carbs: 7g

Protein: 28g

Keto Sausage and Pepper Soup

Serves 6

30 oz. pork sausage

1 tbsp. olive oil

10 oz. raw spinach

1 medium green bell pepper

1 can tomatoes with jalapeños

4 cups beef stock

1 tbsp. onion powder

1 tbsp. chili powder

1 tsp. cumin garlic powder

1 tsp. Italian seasoning

Salt

A delicious low-carb soup that will kill your hunger dead and keep out the cold.

1. In a large pot, heat the olive oil over a medium heat until hot and cook the sausage. Stir.

2. Chop the green pepper and add to the pot. Stir well. Season with salt and pepper. Add the tomatoes and jalapeños. Stir.

3. Add the spinach on top and cover the pot. When it is wilted, incorporate spices and broth and combine.

4. Cover the pot again and let cook for about 30 minutes (heat medium-low). When it is done, remove the lid and let the soup simmer for around 10 minutes.

Nutritional Info per Serving

Calories: 525

Fat: 45g

Net Carbs: 4g

Protein: 28g

Mug Cake with Jalapeño

Serves 1

2 tbsp. almond flour

1 tbsp. flaxseed meal

1 tbsp. butter

1 tbsp. cream cheese

1 egg

1 bacon slice, cooked

½ jalapeño pepper, sliced

½ tsp. baking powder

¼ tsp. salt

Feeling hot, hot, hot? If you like jalapeño peppers, you'll adore this original mug cake.

1. Cook the bacon on a medium heat in a frying pan until crispy.

2. Mix all the ingredients in a container and pour some inside a mug. Microwave for 75 seconds on high.

3. Carefully take out the mug cake out and let cool before eating.

Nutritional Info per Serving

Calories: 430

Fat: 40g

Net Carbs: 4g

Protein: 17g

Fresh Keto Sandwich

SERVES 1

1 cucumber

1 ½ oz. boursin cheese

Meat of your choice, sliced

Make this fresh sandwich with ingredients easily found in your fridge. Put into your Tupperware, cover, and go!

1. Slice the cucumber in half and scoop out the core and seeds with a spoon. Remove the hard outer skin carefully with a knife.

2. In one side place cheese. In the other side fold meat. Place together to form a sandwich!

NUTRITIONAL INFO PER SERVING

Calories: 195

Fat: 14g

Net Carbs: 8g

Protein: 18g

Original Squash Lasagna

SERVES 12

1 lb. spaghetti squash

3 lb. ground beef

30 slices mozzarella cheese

1 large jar marinara sauce

32 oz. whole milk ricotta cheese

You've probably used spaghetti squash to make spaghetti. But have you tried it for lasagna?

1. Cut the spaghetti squash in two halves, placing them face down onto a baking dish. Add a half inch or so of water. Bake for 45 minutes. When finished, carefully pull out the meat of the squash.

2. In a frying pan, cook the ground beef the meat in a pan and add marinara sauce.

3. In a greased baking pan, place a layer of spaghetti squash, cover with the meat sauce, mozzarella and ricotta. Repeat until the pan is full.

4. Bake for 35 minutes at 375°F.

NUTRITIONAL INFO PER SERVING

Calories: 710

Fat: 60g

Net Carbs: 17g

Protein: 45g

Chili Soup

SERVES 8

2 tbsp. butter, unsalted

2 onions

1 pepper

8 chicken thighs (boneless)

8 slices of bacon

1 tsp. thyme

1 tsp. salt

1 tsp. pepper

1 tbsp. garlic, minced

1 tbsp. coconut flour

3 tbsp. lemon juice

1 cup chicken stock

¼ cup unsweetened coconut milk

3 tbsp. tomato paste

Use your crockpot to make this yummy soup, perfect for a chilly day. Get it? Good.

1. Place the butter in the center of the Crock-Pot.

2. Slice the onion and pepper, and add to the Crock-Pot. Then add the chicken thighs. Top with the bacon slices.

3. Season with salt, pepper, minced garlic, and coconut flour. Add the lemon juice, chicken stocks, coconut milk and tomato paste.

4. Cook on low for 6 hours. When it is done, stir and serve.

NUTRITIONAL INFO PER SERVING

Calories: 395

Fat: 20g

Net Carbs: 8g

Protein: 40g

Chicken Nuggets for Keto Nuts

SERVES 4

1 chicken breast, precooked

½ ounce grated parmesan

2 tbsp. almond flour

½ tsp. baking powder

1 egg

1 tbsp. water

These are quick, and healthier than any nuggets you'll ever buy off the shelf! Try them and see for yourself.

1. Cut the chicken breast into slices and then into bite size pieces. Set aside.

2. Combine the parmesan, almond flour, baking powder, and water. Stir.

3. Cover the chicken pieces into the batter, and then place directly into the hot oil. Remove when golden.

NUTRITIONAL INFO PER SERVING

Calories: 165

Fat: 9g

Net Carbs: 3g

Protein: 25g

Cauliflower Rice with Chicken

SERVES 6

4 chicken breasts

1 packet curry paste

1 cup water

3 tbsp. ghee

½ cup heavy cream

1 head cauliflower

Riced cauliflower is a good option when you have to cook for a lot of people. Also, it is low-carb, and when combined with curry chicken, you'll have a great source of protein.

1. In a large pan, melt the ghee, add the curry, and stir. When combined, add the water, and simmer for 5 minutes.

2. Add the chicken, cover and keep cooking for 20 minutes more. When it is done, add the cream and cook for 5 additional minutes.

3. Separately, prepare the cauliflower rice: chop the head into florets and shred. Sauté in a frying pan with a little butter or olive oil, and then turn to low, covering with a lid. Let it steam for 5-8 minutes.

4. Serve along with the chicken curry.

NUTRITIONAL INFO PER SERVING

Calories: 350

Fat: 16g

Net Carbs: 10g

Protein: 40g

Zucchini Keto Wraps

Serves 6

1 zucchini

6 oz. soft goat's cheese

1 tbsp. dried mint

1 tsp. dried dill

Salt and pepper

Oil

This one has to be tried to be believed. It serves up to 6 and the mixture of goat's cheese, mint and dill give it a totally unique twist.

1. Cut off the ends of the zucchini. Slice into ⅛-inch slices and brush with oil. Grill on both sides.

2. Mix together the goat's cheese, mint and dill. Divide into 6 pieces.

3. Wrap the cheese pieces with the zucchini slices and secure with a toothpick.

Nutritional Info per Serving

Calories: 188

Fat: 14g

Net Carbs: 4g

Protein: 15g

Cauliflower Soup with Bacon and Cheddar

Serves 6

1 head of cauliflower

2 tbsp. olive oil

1 medium onion, diced

4 slices bacon

1 tbsp. minced garlic

1 tsp. thyme

12 oz. aged cheddar

1 oz. parmesan cheese

3 cups chicken broth

¼ cup heavy cream

This soup will warm you up on a cold day. The hearty bacon and cheddar flavor makes it one that even picky eaters will gobble right up!

1. Chop the cauliflower, and place on a foil-lined baking sheet. Sprinkle olive oil and season it with salt and pepper. Bake for 35 minutes at 375°F.

2. In a pot, cook the bacon until crispy. Add diced onion and fry it in the bacon grease. When it is tender, add the garlic and the thyme, and cook for 1 minute or less.

3. Incorporate the chicken broth and cauliflower, and simmer, covered, for 20 minutes.

4. Once time is up, blend the ingredients in a food processor or blender until smooth. Place back into the pot. Add the cheddar and the parmesan cheese, and stir until melted.

5. Finally, add the bacon and the double cream, and mix well. If needed, simmer for 10 minutes more, or until heated.

Nutritional Info per Serving

Calories: 340

Fat: 26g

Net Carbs: 10g

Protein: 20g

Keto Casserole with Chicken and Bacon

SERVES 12

12 chicken thighs

1 small onion

4 celery stalks

24 oz. Jimmy Dean sausage

16 oz. sliced mushrooms

16 oz. frozen cauliflower

7 slices bacon

8 oz. shredded cheddar cheese

16 oz. cream cheese, softened

Paprika

This casserole is a complete meal: chicken, bacon, sausage, veggies and cheese will help you stay full of energy for the rest of your day.

1. In the oven, cook the bacon at 400°F for 15 minutes.

2. Meanwhile, dice the chicken and cook in a frying pan. Remove from pan.

3. Brown the sausage. Once it is done, transfer it to the same bowl as the chicken.

4. Chop the onion and celery, and cook them in the remaining sausage grease until translucent.

5. Defrost the cauliflower, and cut the florets into smaller pieces.

6. In a large bowl, add all the ingredients and mix well. Add the cream cheese and mix well.

7. In large pan, place the mixture and sprinkle the paprika.

8. Bake at 350°F for 30 minutes, covered with a foil. Uncover and cook for an additional 10 minutes.

NUTRITIONAL INFO PER SERVING

Calories: 600

Fat: 41g

Net Carbs: 6g

Protein: 53g

Mexican-Style Casserole with Spinach

SERVES 12

1 green pepper

1 onion

20 oz. drained spinach

2 lb. ground pork

2 cans drained diced tomatoes with green chilies

10 tbsp. sour cream

8 oz. mozzarella cheese, shredded

16 oz. cream cheese

4 tsp. taco seasoning

Jalapeños, sliced

This low-carb casserole has all the yummy flavor of tacos, but with a healthier twist.

1. Chop pepper and onion and cook them until translucent. Optional: add diced jalapeños.

2. Place the pepper and onion into a bowl.

3. Cook the spinach by wilting it in a frying pan with a little olive oil. When it is done, add it to the bowl.

4. Cook the ground pork until browned. Season with taco seasoning.

5. Add the diced tomato to the bowl, and incorporate the sour cream, mozzarella and cream cheese. Pour the mixture into a baking dish, and bake at 350°F for 40 minutes.

NUTRITIONAL INFO PER SERVING

Calories: 400

Fat: 30g

Net Carbs: 10g

Protein: 25g

Almond Pizza

SERVES 4

¾ cup almond meal

1½ tsp. baking powder

1½ tsp. granulated sweetener

½ tsp. oregano

¼ tsp. thyme

½ tsp. garlic powder

2 eggs

5 tbsp. butter

½ cup alfredo sauce

4 oz. cheddar cheese

Pizza can be a healthy option when you make the crust with almond meal. Add your favorite toppings and enjoy.

1. Mix the dry ingredients together in a large bowl.

2. Take the eggs (at room temperature) and add to the dry mixture.

3. Melt the butter and incorporate.

4. On a greased pizza pan, spread the crust and pre-cook at 350°F for about 7 minutes.

5. Remove from the oven, and spread the Alfredo Sauce and cheddar cheese on top. Let cook for 5 minutes more.

NUTRITIONAL INFO PER SERVING

Calories: 460

Fat: 45g

Net Carbs: 5g

Protein: 15g

Chicken Salad

Serves 6

4 chicken breasts

1½ cups cream

4½ oz. celery

4 oz. green peppers

1 ounce green onions

¾ cup sugar free sweet relish

¾ cup mayo

3 eggs, hard-boiled

Fresh and nutritious, this easy recipe can be part of a whole meal or served as a side.

1. Place the chicken in an oven-safe pan, and cover it with cream. Cook for 40-60 minutes at 350°F. When it is done, let cool. Discard the liquid.

2. Chop the celery, pepper and onions, and combine them in a bowl. Dice the chicken and add too.

3. Add chopped hardboiled eggs and mix gently.

3. Divide into 6 containers.

Nutritional Info per Serving

Calories: 415

Fat: 24g

Net Carbs: 4g

Protein: 40g

Keto Chicken Thighs

SERVES 6

16 chicken thighs (boneless skinless)

2 cups water

8 oz. cheddar cheese, shredded

24 oz. spinach

Salt and pepper

Garlic powder

Three main ingredients. Thirty minutes. One delicious dinner. You can also divide into containers for a yummy lunch option!

1. Bake the chicken thighs in a covered pan with 2 cups of water at 350°F for 20 minutes. Remove and let cool.

2. Break the chicken into pieces, adding the spinach, cheese, and seasonings.

NUTRITIONAL INFO PER SERVING

Calories: 390

Fat: 25g

Net Carbs: 4g

Protein: 47g

BBQ Chicken Soup

Serves 4

3 medium chicken thighs

2 tsp. chili seasoning

2 tbsp. olive oil

1½ cups chicken broth

1½ cups beef broth

BBQ sauce

¼ cup reduced sugar ketchup

¼ cup tomato paste

2 tbsp. Dijon mustard

1 tbsp. soy sauce

1 tbsp. hot sauce

2½ tsp. liquid smoke

1 tsp. Worcestershire sauce

1½ tsp. garlic powder

1 tsp. onion powder

1 tsp. chili powder

1 tsp. red chili flakes

1 tsp. cumin

¼ cup butter

Salt and pepper

A low-carb soup that comes with an original BBQ flavor. A surefire winner every lunchtime.

1. Take the chicken thighs and de-bone. Reserve the bones. Season with favorite chili seasoning. Bake for 50 minutes at 400°F on a baking tray with foil.

2. In a pot, place olive oil and set on medium high heat. Once it is hot, add the chicken bones. Cook them for 5 minutes and add the broth. Season with salt and pepper.

3. When chicken is done, take off the skin. Incorporate the fat from the chicken into the broth and stir.

4. Make the BBQ Sauce: combine all the already mentioned ingredients for the sauce. Add it to the pot and stir. Let it simmer 20-30 minutes.

5. Emulsify all the fats and liquid together with an immersion blender. Shred the chicken and incorporate into the soup. Cook for 10-20 minutes more.

Nutritional Info per Serving

Calories: 490

Fat: 38g

Net Carbs: 4.5g

Protein: 25g

Keto Pork Stew

Serves 4

1 lb. pork shoulder, cooked and sliced

2 tsp. chili powder

2 tsp. cumin

1 tsp. garlic, minced

½ tsp. salt

½ tsp. pepper

1 tsp. paprika

1 tsp. oregano

¼ tsp. cinnamon

2 bay leaves

6 oz. button mushrooms

½ jalapeño, sliced

½ onion, medium

½ sliced green bell pepper

½ sliced red bell pepper

Juice of ½ a lime

2 cups gelatinous bone broth

2 cups chicken broth

½ cup strong coffee

¼ cup tomato paste

This stew is perfect for when the rain is drizzling down the window outside, and you the family fancies a little pick-me-up.

1. Dice the vegetables, and sauté them in a pan lined with olive oil over high heat. Remove from heat when browned.

2. Chop pork and put into a slow cooker with mushrooms, bone broth, chicken broth and coffee.

3. Incorporate spices and vegetables as well and mix. Place the lid. Cook for 4-10 hours on low.

Nutritional Info per Serving

Calories: 385

Fat: 29g

Net Carbs: 6.4g

Protein: 20g

Keto Enchilada Soup

Serves 4

3 tbsp. olive oil

3 diced celery stalks

1 medium diced red bell pepper

2 tsp. minced garlic

1 cup diced tomatoes

2 tsp. cumin

1 tsp. oregano

1 tsp. chili powder

½ tsp. cayenne pepper

½ cup chopped cilantro

4 cups chicken broth

8 oz. cream cheese

6 oz. shredded chicken

Juice of ½ a lime

This soup is both spicy and creamy, and so delicious that you'll forget all about how healthy it is.

1. In a hot pan with olive oil, sauté the celery and pepper. When the celery starts to become tender, add the tomatoes and cook for 2-3 minutes longer.

2. Incorporate the spices. Add the chicken broth and cilantro, letting it boil. Reduce to a low heat, and simmer for about 20 minutes.

3. Add the cheese and boil again. Reduce to a low heat and simmer for 25 minutes more.

4. Add the shredded chicken with the lime juice. Stir.

5. Season with cilantro and serve.

Nutritional Info per Serving

Calories: 345

Fat: 31g

Net Carbs: 6.3g

Protein: 13g

Grilled Cheese Sandwich

Serves 1

2 eggs

2 tbsp. almond flour

1 ½ tbsp. psyllium husk powder

½ tsp. baking powder

2 tbsp. soft butter

2 oz. cheddar cheese

1 tbsp. butter

A crispy option for lunch, and even better with soup on the side, this little number will have you drooling.

1. Mix the eggs, almond flour, psyllium husk powder, baking powder and butter to make the bun. It should be very thick. Place the mixture into a square container and let it sit to level itself. Microwave for 90 seconds.

2. When it is cooked, remove and slice in half. Place the cheese between the bun, and fry in a pan with melted butter over a medium heat.

Nutritional Info per Serving

Calories: 794

Fat: 72g

Net Carbs: 5g

Protein: 30g

Keto Caprese Salad

SERVES 1

1 tomato

6 oz. fresh mozzarella cheese

¼ cup chopped fresh basil

3 tbsp. olive oil

Freshly cracked black pepper

Salt

This simple recipe takes a quick 5 minutes, but is chock-full of fresh flavor.

1. Put the fresh basil in a food processor with some oil. Blend until it forms a paste.

2. Slice the tomatoes and chop the mozzarella. On the top of each tomato, lay the mozzarella and basil paste. Season with olive oil, black pepper and salt.

NUTRITIONAL INFO PER SERVING

Calories: 407

Fat: 38g

Net Carbs: 3.7g

Protein: 16g

Asian Salad

SERVES 1

1 packet shirataki noodles

2 tbsp. coconut oil

1 cucumber

1 spring onion

¼ tbsp. red pepper flakes

1 tbsp. sesame oil

1 tbsp. rice vinegar

1 tsp. sesame seeds

Salt and pepper

Cucumbers are the fresh tasting stars of this dish. Includes the crunch of fried shirataki noodles, and a slightly spicy flavoring to make it more interesting.

1. Wash the shirataki noodles. Strain off all the excess water. Let them dry on a paper towel.

2. In a pan, heat the coconut oil over a medium-high, and fry the noodles for 5-7 minutes. Remove and set on a paper towel to cool.

3. Peel and slice the cucumber. Arrange on a plate, and add the rest of the ingredients, sprinkling over the cucumber. Let chill for 30 minutes in the fridge.

4. Top with fried shirataki noodles.

NUTRITIONAL INFO PER SERVING

Calories: 418

Fat: 45g

Net Carbs: 8g

Protein: 3g

Vegetarian Curry

SERVES 2

4 tbsp. coconut oil

¼ onion, chopped

1 tsp. garlic, minced

1 cup broccoli florets

Spinach

1 tbsp. red curry paste

½ cup coconut cream (or coconut milk)

2 tsp. soy sauce

1 tsp. ginger

2 tsp. fish sauce

This red curry combines unique flavors and leaves you with an easy recipe that your taste buds will love!

1. On a medium-high heat, add the coconut oil to a pan. Once it is hot, sauté the onions until browned. Add the garlic. Turn to a medium-low heat and add the broccoli. Stir.

2. Once the broccoli is partially cooked, add the curry paste. Let it cook for 1 minute.

3. Add the spinach. When it is cooked, add coconut cream and coconut oil.

3. Mix and add the soy sauce, ginger and fish sauce. Simmer for approximately 10 minutes.

NUTRITIONAL INFO PER SERVING

Calories: 395

Fat: 40g

Net Carbs: 7g

Protein: 6g

Dinners

Keto Pork Chops

Serves 4

½ tsp. peppercorns

1 medium star anise

1 stalk lemongrass

4 halved garlic cloves

4 pork chops (boneless)

1 tbsp. fish sauce

1 tbsp. almond flour

1½ tsp. soy sauce

1 tsp. sesame oil

½ tsp. five spice

½ tbsp. sambal chili paste

½ tbsp. sugar free ketchup

A delicious Asian dinner option with a sumptuous sweet and spicy sauce. This one is guaranteed to be a winner on weekends.

1. Pulverize the peppercorn and star anise (using blender or a mortar).

2. Mix the lemongrass with garlic, fish sauce, soy sauce, sesame oil and five spice powder. Add the powdered peppercorn and star anise. Blend in a food processor until combined.

3. Set the pork on a tray and cover with the mixture on both sides. Cover the tray and marinate for 1-2 hours.

4. Lightly cover each pork chop with almond flour, and pan-fry them at a high temperature. Sear the outsides. Make sure they are done on both sides.

5. Remove and chop into strips.

6. Mix the sambal chili paste and sugar-free ketchup to make the dipping sauce, and serve.

Nutritional Info per Serving

Calories: 224

Fat: 10g

Net Carbs: 5g

Protein: 35g

Original Keto Burger with Portobello Bun

SERVES 1

2 Portobello mushroom caps

½ tbsp. organic extra virgin coconut oil

1 garlic clove

1 tbsp. oregano

6 oz. organic grass fed beef or bison

1 tbsp. Dijon mustard

1 tsp. salt

1 tsp. freshly ground black pepper

¼ cup cheddar cheese

Salt and pepper

Reimagine the burger by knocking up this awesome recipe and enjoy without shame!

1. Clean the Portobello mushrooms, removing the stems and scraping the gills.

2. In a bowl, combine coconut oil with garlic, oregano, salt and pepper. Marinade the Portobello mushrooms in the mixture while you complete the other steps.

3. In a separate bowl, combine the ground meat, mustard, salt, black pepper and cheddar cheese. Form the patties.

4. Place the mushroom caps on a grill for 7-10 minutes. Remove and cook the burgers for 6 minutes on each side.

5. Remove both from the heat and assemble the burger. Add preferred toppings and serve.

NUTRITIONAL INFO PER SERVING

Calories: 730

Fat: 50g

Net Carbs: 5g

Protein: 60g

Pork Hock

Serves 2

1 lb. pork hock

¼ cup rice vinegar

⅓ cup soy sauce

⅓ cup shaoxing cooking wine

¼ cup sweetener

⅓ onion

1 tbsp. butter

Shiitake mushrooms

1 tsp. Chinese five-spice

1 tsp. oregano

2 crushed garlic cloves

A Chinese style recipe. It has all the nutrients needed for your keto diet and will be a frequent dinner on your table.

1. Fry the onions in a frying pan until semi-transparent. Meanwhile, boil the mushrooms until tender.

2. In a third pan, sear the pork hock until browned on all sides.

3. After a few minutes, add all the ingredients in a Crock-Pot and cook for 2 hours on a high heat. Stir, then cook for 2 further hours.

4. Remove the pork and bone it. Slice it and put it back to the pot so that it absorbs more flavor.

5. Serve with the vegetables.

Nutritional Info per Serving

Calories: 550

Fat: 32g

Net Carbs: 20g

Protein: 50g

Keto Crisp Pizza

SERVES 12

8 oz. package of cream cheese (at room temperature)

¼ cup parmesan cheese, grated

2 eggs

1 tsp. garlic powder

½ lb. ground beef

1 chorizo sausage

½ tsp. cumin

¼ tsp. basil

½ tsp. Italian seasoning

¼ tsp. turmeric

Salt and pepper

A low-carb option that can be served either hot or cold and big enough to feed the whole family!

1. Mix cream cheese, parmesan cheese, eggs, pepper and garlic with a hand blender.

2. Grease a baking pan with butter. Spread the dough mixture evenly inside. Cook for 12-15 minutes on the oven at 375°F.

3. Cook the meat in a frying pan and add the spices: cumin, basil, Italian seasoning and turmeric.

4. Once the pizza crust is done, let it cool for 10 minutes, and then cover with tomato sauce and some cheese. Bake for 10 minutes more, and when the cheese starts to melt, add the meat. Broil for 5 minutes more. When it is done, let it cool and slice it up.

NUTRITIONAL INFO PER SERVING

Calories: 145

Fat: 12g

Net Carbs: 1g

Protein: 9g

Meatballs with Bacon and Cheese

Serves 5

1½ lb. ground beef

¾ cup pork rinds, crushed

¾ tsp. salt

¾ tsp. pepper

¾ tsp. cumin

¾ tsp. garlic powder

¾ cup cheddar cheese

4 slices bacon

1 egg

Take meatballs to the next level. These are juicy and taste great. An especially awesome option when you have people over!

1. Process the pork rinds to make a powder.

2. Mix the ground beef, pork rinds, salt, pepper, cumin and garlic powder. Add the cheese and mix well.

3. Cut the bacon into small pieces and fry them in a hot pan until they reach the desired doneness. Let them cool. Add the bacon to the meat and combine well.

4. Form the meatballs.

3. Cook the meatballs in a pan, browning them on all sides, then cover with a lid for 10 minutes. When finished, let them sit for 5 minutes or so before enjoying. Top with the sauce of your choice.

Nutritional Info per Serving

Calories: 450

Fat: 26g

Net Carbs: 3g

Protein: 50g

Bacon Wrapped Chicken

SERVES 4

2 skinless chicken breasts, boneless

2 oz. blue cheese

4 slices ham

8 slices bacon

A simple recipe with chicken and bacon, sure to go down as a winner in everyone's book. It's easy to make it and absolutely stacked with protein.

1. Slice the breast halves in half lengthwise.

2. Lay out 2 slices of ham, and place a line of cheese in the middle. Roll up, and place inside the chicken breast.

3. Wrap the chicken breast with 4 slices of bacon, covering the entire breast.

4. Place the breasts in an oven-proof skillet (greased with butter or coconut oil), and brown the bacon all over. Remove from the skillet and place in the oven to cook for 45 minutes at 325°F. Let sit for 10 minutes before serving.

NUTRITIONAL INFO PER SERVING

Calories: 270

Fat: 11g

Net Carbs: 0.50g

Protein: 38g

Keto Broccoli Soup

SERVES 4

1 head broccoli

¼ cup heavy cream

¼ cup cream cheese

¼ cup sour cream

¼ cup almond milk

4 oz. cheddar cheese

½ onion

½ chicken bouillon cube

You can probably find all the ingredients for this one in your fridge already, so knock it up and enjoy!

1. Remove the florets from the broccoli. Steam them on the stove.

2. Put the florets into a blender and add the rest of the ingredients. Blend until the mixture reaches the desired consistency.

3. Pour into a pot and simmer until heated (10 minutes or so).

NUTRITIONAL INFO PER SERVING

Calories: 270

Fat: 25g

Net Carbs: 8g

Protein: 10g

Little Portobello Pizza

SERVES 1

3 Portobello mushrooms

Olive oil

3 tsp. pizza seasoning

3 tomato slices

9 spinach leaves

1½ oz. mozzarella

1½ oz. Monterey jack

1½ oz. cheddar cheese

12 pepperoni slices

These little pizzas are made from Portobello caps. An original way to finish your day and keep those cravings in check.

1. Prepare the Portobello mushrooms by washing them, removing both the gills and the stems.

2. Sprinkle with olive oil and pizza seasoning, and then top with all the other ingredients, except the pepperoni slices.

3. Cook at 450°F for 6 minutes. Add the pepperoni slices and broil until crispy.

NUTRITIONAL INFO PER SERVING

Calories: 275

Fat: 20g

Net Carbs: 5g

Protein: 20g

Bacon Wrap

SERVES 4

16 oz. beef

Montreal steak seasoning

4 bacon slices

Delicious, packed with protein and ready to roll nice and fast. What's not to love?

1. Cut the beef into cubes and season it.

2. Cut the bacon slices in four.

3. Wrap the beef with the bacon, and pierce with a toothpick. Repeat 2 or 3 times. Fry for 3 minutes.

NUTRITIONAL INFO PER SERVING

Calories: 217

Fat: 10g

Net Carbs: 0g

Protein: 30g

Cheddar Biscuits

SERVES 1

2 cups Carbquik

2 oz. unsalted butter, cold

4 oz. shredded cheddar cheese

½ tsp. garlic powder

½ tsp. salt

¼ cup heavy cream

¼ cup water

We adore our cheddar biscuits. Stuff them with your favorite fillings, or have them as a side to your favorite dinner dish.

1. In a bowl, mix Carbquik and add the cold butter. Cut in the pieces of butter until the mixture has little balls of butter and flour about the size of peas. Add the cheese, garlic powder and salt and combine together.

2. Add the heavy cream and water. Mix until a dough forms. Separate them into 6 pieces and place on a greased sheet. Bake them at 450°F for about 8-10 minutes.

NUTRITIONAL INFO PER SERVING

Calories: 45

Fat: 4g

Net Carbs: 2.5g

Protein: 1.6g

Sausage & Cabbage Skillet Melt

SERVES 4

4 spicy Italian chicken sausages

1½ cups green cabbage, shredded

1½ cups purple cabbage, shredded

½ cup onion, diced

2 tsp. coconut oil

2 slices Colby jack cheese

2 tsp. fresh cilantro, chopped

Mildly spicy, super satisfying and perfect for a keto dinner. Try this one out with company.

1. Shred the cabbage (or use pre-shredded cabbage) and chop the onion.

2. Melt the coconut oil, and fry the onion and cabbage in a large skillet. Turn to medium-high and cook for 8 minutes.

3. Add the sausage, and stir to mix it into the vegetables. Cook for 8 further minutes.

4. Add the cheese on top and cover.

5. Turn off the heat and wait while the cheese melts into the vegetables.

NUTRITIONAL INFO PER SERVING

Calories: 233

Fat: 15g

Net Carbs: 5g

Protein: 20g

Keto Chicken Tikka Masala

Serves 5

1 lb. chicken thighs (boneless/skinless)

2 tbsp. olive oil

2 tsp. onion powder

3 minced garlic cloves

1 inch grated ginger root

3 tbsp. tomato paste

5 tsp. garam masala

2 tsp. smoked paprika

4 tsp. kosher salt

10 oz. diced tomatoes (can)

1 cup heavy cream

1 cup coconut milk

Fresh chopped cilantro

1 tsp. guar gum

Chicken Tikka Masala is a super flavorful and delicious curry that you can now make keto style!

1. De-bone the chicken thighs. Chop the chicken into bite-sized pieces.

2. In a slow cooker, add the chicken and grate the ginger on top.

3. In another bowl, mix the tomato paste and canned tomatoes with the rest of the dry spices. Add ½ cup coconut milk and stir. Add to the slow cooker.

3. Cook on low for 6 hours or on high for 3 hours.

4. Once finished, add the remaining coconut milk, double cream, and guar gum. Mix.

Nutritional Info per Serving

Calories: 495

Fat: 43g

Net Carbs: 5g

Protein: 25g

Spaghetti Squash with Meat Sauce

Serves 8

2 spaghetti squashes

2 lb. ground beef

33-oz. jar of spaghetti sauce

1 tbsp. minced garlic

1 tbsp. Italian seasoning

Parmesan cheese

It's not even funny how easy this is - and it's just as good as the real thing!

1. Cut the spaghetti squash in half and scrape out the guts. Cook the remaining shell and meat in a glass container partially filled with water at 375°F for 45 minutes or until soft.

2. Brown some beef on the stove. Add the seasonings, the sauce, and mix. Heat through.

3. Carefully remove the cooked spaghetti squash from the oven, and use a fork to create the spaghetti. Serve with the sauce.

Nutritional Info per Serving

Calories: 170

Fat: 15g

Net Carbs: 12g

Protein: 11g

Keto Guacamole

SERVES 8

4 avocados

1 small onion, chopped

2 tomatoes, chopped

1 jalapeño, chopped

1 tbsp. lime juice

½ tsp. salt

½ tsp. cumin

½ tsp. salt

½ tsp. cayenne pepper

1 tbsp. minced garlic

No recipe book is compete without guacamole, and we've got the perfect keto mix right here.

1. In a large bowl, add the chopped and peeled avocados and the lime juice. Mash the avocados with a potato masher and add spices.

2. Add the jalapeños, onions and tomatoes and mix again.

3. Let rest for an hour before serving.

NUTRITIONAL INFO PER SERVING

Calories: 141

Fat: 11g

Net Carbs: 12g

Protein: 4g

Cheesy Bacon Brussels Sprouts

Serves 4

5 slices bacon

16 oz. Brussels sprouts

6 oz. cheddar cheese

The combination of cheese and bacon transform this much maligned vegetable into everybody's new best friend!

1. Fry the bacon until crisp. Cut into small pieces.

2. Shred the Brussels sprouts with a food processor. In the bacon grease, fry them until tender.

3. Add in the bacon and cheese when the Brussels sprouts are crispy and translucent.

4. Cook until melted.

Nutritional Info per Serving

Calories: 260

Fat: 22g

Net Carbs: 5g

Protein: 17g

Keto Parmesan Chicken

SERVES 4

For the Chicken:
3 chicken breasts
1 cup mozzarella cheese
Salt and pepper

For the Coating:
2½ oz. pork rinds
¼ cup flaxseed meal
½ cup parmesan cheese
1 tsp. oregano
½ tsp. salt
½ tsp. pepper
¼ tsp. red pepper flakes
½ tsp. garlic
2 tsp. paprika
1 egg
1½ tsp. chicken broth
The Sauce
¼ cup olive oil
1 cup tomato sauce
½ tsp. garlic
½ tsp. oregano
Salt and pepper

A keto twist on the traditional Italian dish that will make your mouth water and your stomach purr with satisfaction.

1. In a food processor, grind up the pork rinds, parmesan cheese and spices.

2. Slice the chicken breasts into thirds, and season them with salt and pepper.

3. In another bowl, make the coating: whisk eggs and add the chicken broth.

4. Begin to make the sauce by combining all the sauce ingredients in a saucepan and whisking. Let simmer for 20 minutes.

5. Bread the chicken slices: dip them into the egg mixture and then into the pork rind coating. Place on a piece of foil.

6. In a pan, heat a few tbsp. of olive oil and fry the chicken. Place the fried chicken into a casserole dish, cover with sauce and cheese. Bake for 10 minutes at 400ñF.

NUTRITIONAL INFO PER SERVING

Calories: 646
Fat: 47g
Net Carbs: 5g
Protein: 49g

Creamy Chicken

Serves 1

5 oz. chicken breast

1 tbsp. olive oil

3 oz. mushrooms

¼ small onion, sliced

½ cup chicken broth

¼ cup heavy cream

½ tsp. dried tarragon

1 tsp. grain mustard

Salt and pepper

A unique recipe that will make a special dinner. Chicken is always a good source of fats and proteins.

1. Cut the chicken into cubes, season them, and brown with olive oil. Remove and place on a plate.

2. Add mushrooms to the same pan and cook until browned. Add the onion and cook until the onion is translucent.

3. Add the chicken broth. Reduce by letting it boil for 3-5 minutes.

4. Add the rest of the ingredients and seasonings, and mix. Add the chicken, and let it simmer 3-5 more minutes.

Nutritional Info per Serving

Calories: 489

Fat: 43g

Net Carbs: 5g

Protein: 30g

Cheeseburger Soup with Bacon

SERVES 5

5 slices bacon

12 oz. ground beef

2 tbsp. butter

3 cups beef broth

½ tsp. garlic powder

½ tsp. onion powder

2 tsp. brown mustard

½ tsp. red pepper flakes

1 tsp. chili powder

1 tsp. cumin

2½ tsp. tomato paste

1 medium dill pickle, diced

1 cup shredded cheddar cheese

3 ounce cream cheese

½ cup heavy cream

1½ tsp. salt

½ tsp. black pepper

Cheeseburger soup? With bacon? Yeah, you're just going to have to trust us on this one.

1. Cook the bacon in a frying pan until crispy. Remove and crumble into a small bowl.

2. In the leftover bacon fat, brown the ground beef.

3. Transfer the meat into a soup pot, adding both butter and spices. Let the butter melt.

4. Incorporate beef broth, tomato paste, cheese and pickles and cook until melted. Cover the pot, turn to low heat and simmer for 20 minutes more.

5. Turn the stove off, and add the double cream and crumbled bacon. Mix well.

NUTRITIONAL INFO PER SERVING

Calories: 573

Fat: 48g

Net Carbs: 4g

Protein: 24g

Low Carb Chicken Nuggets

SERVES 4

For the Nuggets:

24 oz. chicken thighs

1 egg

For the Crust:

1½ oz. pork rinds

¼ cup flax meal

¼ cup almond meal

Zest of 1 lime

⅛ tsp. garlic powder

¼ tsp. paprika

¼ tsp. chili powder

⅛ tsp. onion powder

⅛ tsp. cayenne pepper

¼ tsp. salt

¼ tsp. pepper

For the Sauce:

½ cup mayonnaise

½ avocado

¼ tsp. garlic powder

1 tbsp. lime juice

⅛ tsp. cumin

½ tsp. red chili flakes

This is a different take on the traditional nugget, but you may just end up loving it even more.

1. Dry the chicken and cut into bite-size pieces.

2. Put all the crust ingredients into a food processor and mix.

3. In a bowl place the crumbs and a whisked egg in a different one. Dip the chicken into the egg, the crust and then lay on a greased baking sheet. Bake for 15-20 minutes at 400°F.

4. To make the sauce, just mix all the sauce ingredients together.

NUTRITIONAL INFO PER SERVING

Calories: 615

Fat: 53g

Net Carbs: 2g

Protein: 39g

Keto Salad with Radish and Asparagus

Serves 4

1½ lb. asparagus spears

10 radishes

4 oz. sour cream

1 tbsp. lemon juice

1 tsp. white wine vinegar

1 tbsp. dill

1 tbsp. mayonnaise

1 tbsp. olive oil

1 tsp. parsley

Pepper

This salad goes well with your favorite grilled chicken, fish or meat, but it can also make a whole meal by itself if you're feeling light and fresh.

1. Boil the water in a pot with a dash of salt. Wash the asparagus stalks and cut off the woody ends. Add to the pot and boil for 2-3 minutes or until desired softness.

2. Place the asparagus into a pot of ice water to stop the cooking process.

3. Cut the tops and bottoms off the radishes and slice them thinly.

4. Make the dressing by blending the rest of the ingredients.

5. Mix the dressing, radishes, and asparagus together until evenly coated.

Nutritional Info per Serving

Calories: 156

Fat: 10g

Net Carbs: 10g

Protein: 5g

Sushi!

Serves 3

16 oz. cauliflower

6 oz. softened cream cheese

1-2 tbsp. unseasoned rice vinegar

1 tbsp. soy sauce

5 sheets nori

1-½-inch length of cucumber

½ avocado

5 oz. smoked salmon

You won't believe it: sushi for your keto diet! Here is a simple recipe you can use for movie nights with family and friends.

1. Rice the cauliflower with a food processor.

2. Cut each cucumber into thin lengthwise slices. Keep in the fridge until ready.

3. Cook the cauliflower rice in a hot pan until almost tender. Season with soy sauce. When it is done, mix in a bowl with cream cheese and rice vinegar, and set in the fridge until cool.

4. Thinly slice the avocado.

5. Place a nori sheet on a bamboo roller. Spread some of the cauliflower over the nori sheet to almost cover. Layer the cucumber, avocado and salmon on one end. Roll tightly.

Nutritional Info per Serving

Calories: 350

Fat: 26g

Net Carbs: 6g

Protein: 18g

Kung Pao Chicken

Serves 3

For the Chicken:

2 medium chicken thighs

1 tsp. ground ginger

¼ cup peanuts

½ green pepper

4 de-seeded red bird's eye chilies

2 large spring onions

Salt and pepper

For the Sauce:

1 tbsp. soy sauce

2 tbsp. chili garlic paste

2 tsp. rice wine vinegar

1 tbsp. reduced-sugar ketchup

½ tsp. maple extract

2 tsp. sesame oil

10 drops liquid stevia

Asian food for dinner is always a great option. This dish tastes amazing and is super easy to make. The combination of peanuts and chicken give it a keto kick.

1. Cut the chicken into small pieces and season with salt, pepper and ginger.

2. Cook the chicken in a pan over a medium-high heat until browned (approximately 10 minutes).

3. Make the sauce by combining all the sauce ingredients.

4. Chop the vegetables and chilies. When the chicken is done, add all the ingredients and cook for 3-4 minutes longer. Add the sauce and let it boil until reduced.

Nutritional Info per Serving

Calories: 360

Fat: 27.5g

Net Carbs: 3g

Protein: 22g

Stuffed Burgers

SERVES 2

8 oz. ground beef

1 tsp. salt

½ tsp. pepper

1 tsp. Cajun seasoning

1 ounce mozzarella cheese

2 oz. cheddar cheese

1 tbsp. butter

2 slices pre-cooked bacon

These stuffed burgers are so delicious. You can make them on the grill, or even in the oven if the weather isn't on your side.

1. Take the ground beef and season it with salt, pepper and Cajun seasoning. Flatten into a patty and place mozzarella cheese inside. Cover and flatten again.

2. In a pan, heat the butter (1 tbsp. per burger). Then add the burger, cooking for 2-3 minutes on each side. Top with cheese, cover with a lid and let steam for 2 minutes more.

3. Slice the bacon slices in half and place on top.

NUTRITIONAL INFO PER SERVING

Calories: 615

Fat: 50g

Net Carbs: 1.5g

Protein: 35g

Keto Totchos

SERVES 2

2 servings keto tater tots

6 oz. ground beef

2 oz. shredded cheddar cheese

2 tbsp. sour cream

6 sliced black olives

1 tbsp. salsa

½ jalapeño pepper, sliced

Totchos are crisp tater tots dressed like nachos and topped with sour cream, salsa and jalapeños. Using keto tater tots, this recipe will fulfill your every craving.

1. In a small casserole pan, place 9-10 keto tots and add half of the ground beef and half of the cheese. Place a second layer of tots, and add the rest of the meat and cheese.

2. Broil in the oven for 5 minutes until the cheese melts, and serve with sour cream, black olives, salsa and jalapeño.

NUTRITIONAL INFO PER SERVING

Calories: 638

Fat: 53g

Net Carbs: 6g

Protein: 32g

Keto Thai Zoodles

SERVES 1

3½ oz. chicken thighs

½ tsp. curry powder

3½ oz. zucchini

1 stalk spring onion

1 clove garlic

1 tsp. soy sauce

½ tsp. oyster sauce

⅛ tsp. white pepper

1 tbsp. butter

1 tbsp. coconut oil

1 egg

1⅕ oz. bean sprouts

1 tsp. lime juice

Chopped red chilies

Salt and pepper

A dish all the way from Asia is now available on your dinner table in keto form!

1. Marinate the chicken with curry powder, salt and pepper.
2. Make the zoodles out of the zucchini by slicing it into very thin strips. Chop the onion and garlic into small pieces.
3. Make the sauce by mixing the soy sauce, oyster sauce and white pepper.
4. Cook the chicken with the butter until they are browned and cut into bit-sized pieces.
5. In the same pan on high heat, add coconut oil and sauté the onion and the garlic. Add the egg and cook until slightly browned.
6. Add in the bean sprouts and zoodles, and mix. Pour in the sauce, add the chicken, and stir.
7. Garnish with some chopped red chillies and lemon juice.

NUTRITIONAL INFO PER SERVING

Calories: 581

Fat: 50g

Net Carbs: 7g

Protein: 26g

Pork Pies

SERVES 4

1 lb. ground pork

4 tbsp. grated parmesan cheese

2 beaten eggs

½ tsp. ground nutmeg

½ tsp. ginger

½ tsp. cardamom

½ lemon zest

4 tart shells (keto)

Salt and pepper

This amazing recipe with Irish roots is a great dinner choice when you need something simple and hearty.

1. In a pan over a high heat, place the meat and spices. When it is slightly cooked, remove and add the egg and lemon.

2. Put some of the mixture into keto pie shells and bake for about 20-25 minutes. Remove from oven and let cool.

NUTRITIONAL INFO PER SERVING

Calories: 560

Fat: 23g

Net Carbs: 6g

Protein: 30g

Stuffed Peppers

Serves 1

4 poblano peppers

1 lb. ground pork

1 tbsp. bacon fat

1 tsp. cumin

1 tsp. chili powder

½ onion

1 tomato

7 baby bella mushrooms

¼ cup packed cilantro

Salt and pepper

This easy recipe includes a delicious combination of vegetables, mushrooms and pork. Stuffed pepper never tasted so good!

1. In the oven, broil the poblano peppers for approximately 8-10 minutes.

2. Brown the pork in bacon fat. Season with salt, pepper, cumin and chili.

3. Incorporate the diced onion and minced garlic. Mix everything together and add the sliced mushrooms. Once they absorb all the fat in the pan, add the chopped cilantro and tomato. Cook for 12 minutes.

4. Put the mixture into the peppers, and bake for 8 minutes at 350°F.

Nutritional Info per Serving

Calories: 368

Fat: 27g

Net Carbs: 6g

Protein: 22g

Chicken Satay

Serves 3

1 lb. ground chicken

4 tbsp. soy sauce

3 tbsp. peanut butter

1 tbsp. erythritol

1 tbsp. rice vinegar

2 tsp. sesame oil

2 tsp. chili paste

1 tsp. minced garlic

¼ tsp. cayenne

¼ tsp. paprika

½ tsp. lime juice

2 chopped spring onions

⅓ sliced yellow pepper

This is a low-carb dish that is easy, tasty, and different. Your whole family will love it.

1. In a pan over a medium-high heat, put the sesame oil and sauté the ground chicken. Add the rest of the ingredients and mix well.

2. When it is cooked, add the onions and yellow pepper, mix, and enjoy.

Nutritional Info per Serving

Calories: 395

Fat: 24g

Net Carbs: 4g

Protein: 35g

Glazed Salmon

Serves 2

10 oz. salmon filet

2 tbsp. soy sauce

2 tsp. sesame oil

1 tbsp. rice vinegar

1 tsp. ginger, minced

2 tsp. garlic minced

1 tbsp. red boat fish sauce

1 tbsp. sugar free ketchup

2 tbsp. white wine

Salmon is an excellent source of Omega 3 fats, which are key in your keto diet. You'll enjoy this one just as much as your body does.

1. In a container, add all the ingredients (except for the ketchup, sesame oil and white wine) and marinate the salmon in them for 10-15 minutes.

2. In a pan over high heat bring add sesame oil to smoke point and place the filet in, skin side down.

3. Cook until crisp on both sides (4 minutes per side). Remove the fish to make the glaze.

4. Add ketchup and white wine to the marinade. Put in the pan and simmer for 5 minutes, or until reduced to a glaze.

Nutritional Info per Serving

Calories: 372

Fat: 24g

Net Carbs: 3g

Protein: 35g

Coconut Shrimp

SERVES 3

For the Coconut Shrimp:

1 lb. peeled and de-veined shrimp

2 egg whites

1 cup unsweetened coconut flakes

2 tbsp. coconut flour

For the Sweet Chili Dipping Sauce:

½ cup sugar free apricot preserves

1 ½ tsp. rice wine vinegar

1 tbsp. lime juice

1 medium diced red chili

¼ tsp. red pepper flakes

A traditional recipe turned low-carb. And don't worry, it's still crispy and delicious!

1. Beat the egg whites until they form soft peaks. Prepare two separate bowls with coconut flakes and coconut flour.

2. Dip the shrimp and in coconut flour, then egg whites, and then coconut flakes. Place the shrimp onto a greased baking sheet. Bake at 400°F for 15 minutes. Flip and broil for 3-5 minutes, or until browned and crispy.

3. Make the sauce by mixing all the ingredients for the dipping sauce.

NUTRITIONAL INFO PER SERVING

Calories: 398

Fat: 22g

Net Carbs: 7g

Protein: 36g

Desserts

Keto Pavlova

SERVES 6

For the Base:

4 egg whites

½ cup erythritol

1 tsp. vanilla extract

1 tsp. lemon juice

2 tsp. xanthan gum

For the Filling:

1 cup heavy cream

3 oz. frozen berries

For the Topping:

18 fresh raspberries

1-2 mint leaves

This dessert is partially frozen, and perfect for that satiating that sweet craving.

1. Separate the egg white from the yolk, and whisk the egg whites. Add erythritol while beating and continue beating until stiff peaks form.

2. Carefully fold in the vanilla extract, lemon juice and xanthan gum. Fold together with a silicone spatula.

3. Place parchment paper on a baking sheet. Using a pencil, outline a cup as a guide for where to spread the mixture. Spoon the batter into the paper, then make a small hole in the middle.

4. Bake for 1 hour at 300°F.

5. Make the filling by blending the frozen berries with heavy cream for approximately 3 minutes, or until a thick, creamy consistency is achieved.

5. When the pavlovas are done, spoon the berry sauce inside, and top with fresh raspberries and mint leaves.

NUTRITIONAL INFO PER SERVING

Calories: 163

Fat: 16g

Net Carbs: 2.5g

Protein: 3g

Amaretti Cookies

SERVES 16 COOKIES

1 cup almond flour

2 tbsp. coconut flour

½ tsp. baking powder

¼ tsp. cinnamon

½ tsp. salt

½ cup erythritol

2 eggs

4 tbsp. coconut oil

½ tsp. vanilla extract

½ tsp. almond extract

2 tbsp. sugar-free jam

1 tbsp. coconut, shredded

These cookies are easy to make and can feed a mini horde. Or just you, for a few days!

1. Combine all the dry ingredients.

2. Add the wet ingredients. Mix well.

3. In a parchment paper lined on a baking sheet, form the cookies. Make a dent in the middle of each one of them. Bake at 400°F for about 16 minutes. Let them cool.

4. Add in each indent a little bit of jam, and top with a sprinkle of shredded coconut.

NUTRITIONAL INFO PER SERVING

Calories: 86

Fat: 8g

Net Carbs: 1g

Protein: 2.5g

Pumpkin Ice Cream with Pecans

Serves 4

½ cup toasted and chopped pecans

2 tbsp. salted butter

½ cup cottage cheese

½ cup pumpkin puree

1 tsp. pumpkin spice

2 cups coconut milk

3 egg yolks

½ tsp. xanthan gum

⅓ cup erythritol

20 drops liquid stevia

1 tsp. maple extract

Two classic flavors are combined into one in this yummy recipe, perfect for fall evenings.

1. Roast the butter and pecans in a saucepan for 8-10 minutes.

2. Blend together the rest of the ingredients using an immersion blender.

3. Add the mixture to an ice cream machine, adding the pecans and butter on top.

4. Follow the instructions of the machine, and enjoy.

Nutritional Info per Serving

Calories: 250

Fat: 22g

Net Carbs: 4g

Protein: 7g

Peanut Butter Bar

SERVES 8

For the Crust:

1 cup almond flour

¼ melted cup butter

½ tsp. cinnamon

1 tbsp. erythritol

Salt

For the Fudge:

¼ cup heavy cream

¼ cup melted butter

½ cup peanut butter

¼ cup erythritol

½ tsp. vanilla extract

⅛ tsp. xanthan gum

For the Topping:

⅓ cup chopped vegan dark chocolate

It's easy to make, and even easier to eat – be careful or you'll develop a peanut butter addiction!

1. Combine the almond flour, erythritol, cinnamon and salt with half of the melted butter.

2. Pack the mixture into a baking dish lined with parchment paper. Bake for 10 minutes and let cool.

3. Blend the fudge ingredients together.

4. Spread the mix over the crust and add the chopped chocolate on top.

5. Place in the fridge and freeze for 1-2 hours.

NUTRITIONAL INFO PER SERVING

Calories: 300

Fat: 20g

Net Carbs: 3g

Protein: 5g

Strawberry and Cream Cakes

Serves 5

For the Mix:

3 eggs

3 oz. cream cheese

¼ tsp. baking powder

½ tsp. vanilla extract

2 tbsp. erythritol

For the Filling:

10 strawberries

1 cup heavy cream

A light, fluffy cake perfect for a summer barbeque or as a light dessert.

1. Separate the eggs. Whisk the egg whites until stiff peaks form. In another bowl, add the egg yolks, the cream cheese, baking powder, vanilla extract and the erythritol and combine until smooth.

2. Gently incorporate the egg white mix into the egg yolk mix by folding. Form the mixture into small cake shapes on a baking sheet covered with parchment paper.

3. Whip the heavy cream until thick.

3. Bake at 300°F for 25-30 minutes. Let them cool. Cut them open and place strawberries and cream inside.

Nutritional Info per Serving

Calories: 275

Fat: 30g

Net Carbs: 3.7g

Protein: 6g

Chocolate Macaroon Cookies with Coconut

Serves 20

1 cup almond flour

3 tbsp. coconut flour

¼ cup cocoa powder

½ tsp. baking powder

⅓ cup erythritol

⅓ cup unsweetened coconut, shredded

¼ tsp. salt

2 eggs (at room temperature)

¼ cup coconut oil

1 tsp. vanilla extract

These amazing cookies are super low-carb! They are soft inside but with a crunchy shell.

1. Combine all the dry ingredients. Add the wet ingredients and mix well.

2. Roll the dough into small balls.

3. On a lined baking sheet, place the dough balls a few inches apart and bake for 15-20 minutes at 350°F.

4. Sprinkle with shredded coconut.

Nutritional Info per Serving

Calories: 77

Fat: 7g

Net Carbs: 1g

Protein: 2.2g

Keto Covered Macaroons

SERVES 12

1 cup unsweetened shredded coconut

1 egg white

¼ cup erythritol

½ tsp. almond extract

1 ounce sugar-free chocolate

2 tbsp. coconut oil

Salt

Are they cookies or are they fat bombs? Both!

1. Bake coconut on parchment paper lined baking sheet at 350°F for 5 minutes or until toasted.

2. Beat the egg until it doubles in size. Incorporate erythritol, salt and almond extract little by little, while continuing to mix.

3. Add the toasted coconut and mix well.

4. Pack little balls of the mixture into a 1½" ice cream scoop, then place them on a parchment paper lined baking sheet. Bake for 15 minutes at 350°F.

5. Melt the chocolate together with the coconut oil. You can do this in the microwave: heat for 10-second intervals until melted.

6. When the macaroons are done, drizzle each one of them with the chocolate.

NUTRITIONAL INFO PER SERVING

Calories: 75

Fat: 7g

Net Carbs: 1g

Protein: 1g

Poppy Seed Soufflés

SERVES 4

2 separated large eggs

¼ cup erythritol

1 cup whole milk ricotta

2 tsp. lemon zest

1 tbsp. lemon juice

1 tsp. vanilla extract

1 tsp. poppy seeds

These soufflés are low-carb, and the delicate lemon poppy seed flavor provides a slightly different twist to one of our favorite staples.

1. Whisk the egg whites until foamy. Add erythritol and beat until stiff peaks form.

2. Mix the egg yolks with ricotta cheese and erythritol. Add the lemon zest and juice.

3. Incorporate the extract and poppy seed and mix well.

4. Add the egg white into the mixture by carefully folding.

5. Divide the batter into 4 small ramekins and bake at 375°F for about 20 minutes. Take care not to open the oven until they are finished or they may collapse.

NUTRITIONAL INFO PER SERVING

Calories: 150

Fat: 10g

Net Carbs: 3g

Protein: 10g

Keto Choc Tarts

SERVES 4

For the Crust:

¼ cup flaxseed meal

2 tbsp. almond flour

1 tbsp. erythritol

1 egg white

For the Top Layer:

Avocado

4 tbsp. cocoa powder

¼ cup erythritol

½ tsp. vanilla extract

½ tsp. cinnamon

2 tbsp. heavy cream

For the Middle Layer:

4 tbsp. peanut butter

2 tbsp. butter

Chocolate and peanut butter are mixed together in this amazingly moreish keto recipe.

1. Make the crust by pulverizing the flaxseed until the mixture is mealy. Add the rest of the crust ingredients and mix well.

2. Place the crust inside tart pans making sure to press them to the bottom. Get the sides up. Bake at 350°F for 8 minutes. Remove and let them cool.

3. In a small blender, combine all the top layer ingredients until smooth.

4. Melt the peanut butter with the butter in the microwave to make the middle layer.

5. Pour the middle layer mixture onto the tarts and place in the fridge for 30 minutes or until it is set. When it is done, add the top layer. Place in the fridge for 30 more minutes.

NUTRITIONAL INFO PER SERVING

Calories: 300

Fat: 27g

Net Carbs: 4g

Protein: 10g

Easy Pumpkin Pie Cheesecake

Serves 8

For the Crust:

¾ cup almond flour

½ cup flaxseed meal

½ cup butter

1 tsp. pumpkin pie spice

25 drops liquid stevia

For the Filling:

4 oz. cream cheese

⅓ cup pumpkin puree

2 tbsp. sour cream

¼ cup heavy cream

3 tbsp. butter

¼ tsp. pumpkin pie spice

25 drops liquid stevia

This yummy cheesecake doesn't even need to bake. It's the perfect creamy dessert after a Thanksgiving dinner!

1. Combine all the dry ingredients for the crust and add the butter and stevia. Mix.

2. Place some dough into a tart pan and press it to the bottom.

3. Mix all the filling ingredients and blend with an immersion blender.

4. Pour the filling into crusts and refrigerate for 4 hours. Top with whipped cream if desired.

Nutritional Info per Serving

Calories: 267

Fat: 25g

Net Carbs: 4g

Protein: 6g

Chia Bars

SERVES 14

½ cup almonds, toasted

1 tbsp. + 1 tsp. coconut oil

4 tbsp. erythritol

2 tbsp. butter

¼ cup heavy cream

¼ tsp. liquid stevia

1½ tsp. vanilla extract

½ cup coconut flakes, unsweetened and shredded

¼ cup chia seeds

½ cup coconut cream

2 tbsp. coconut flour

High in fats and low on carbs, these are a nice twist on the traditional fat bomb.

1. In a food processor, blend the toasted almonds until crumbly. Add 1 tbsp. of coconut oil and 2 tbsp. of erythritol. Process until it becomes almond butter.

2. In a pan, heat the butter, and add heavy cream, stevia, erythritol and vanilla. Mix together until they are a bubbly mixture. Add the almond butter and stir.

3. Grind chia seed in a blender to form a powdery mix. In a separate pan, toast the chia seeds and coconut flakes.

4. Combine all the ingredients together, and add coconut cream (previously melted), coconut oil and coconut flour. Mix and place into any pan. Refrigerate for 1 hour, cut into small squares, and refrigerate again for a couple of hours.

NUTRITIONAL INFO PER SERVING

Calories: 121

Fat: 11g

Net Carbs: 1.5g

Protein: 2.5g

Avocado Ice Cream with Chocolate

SERVES 6

2 avocados

1 cup coconut milk

½ cup heavy cream

½ cup cocoa powder

2 tsp. vanilla extract

½ cup powdered erythritol

25 drops liquid stevia

6 squares unsweetened baking chocolate

This original avocado ice cream also has an exciting chocolate element that will go down a treat with friends and family.

1. In a bowl, add avocado, coconut milk, cream and vanilla extract. Mix with an immersion blender until smooth.

2. Add the powdered erythritol, stevia and cocoa powder. Mix well.

3. Break the baking chocolate and incorporate to the mixture.

4. Place in the fridge for 6-12 hours. Remove 20 minutes before serving and add the mixture to the ice cream machine, following the manufacturer's instructions.

NUTRITIONAL INFO PER SERVING

Calories: 240

Fat: 22g

Net Carbs: 4g

Protein: 4g

Chocolate Roll Cake

SERVES 12

For the Mix:

1 cup almond flour

4 tbsp. melted butter

3 eggs

¼ cup psyllium husk powder

¼ cup cocoa powder

¼ cup coconut milk

¼ cup sour cream

¼ cup erythritol

1 tsp. vanilla

1 tsp. baking powder

For the Filling:

8 oz. cream cheese

8 tbsp. butter

¼ cup sour cream

¼ cup erythritol

¼ tsp. stevia

1 tsp. vanilla

With a rich chocolate cake and a yummy cream cheese filling, this cake roll will kick your cravings to the curb in style.

1. In a bowl, combine all the dry ingredients and slowly add the wet ingredients, mixing well.

2. Spread the dough onto a parchment paper covered cookie sheet. Bake at 350°F for 12-15 minutes.

3. Make the filling by mixing all the ingredients together. When the cake is done, spread the filling over it and roll cake tightly.

NUTRITIONAL INFO PER SERVING

Calories: 275

Fat: 25g

Net Carbs: 3g

Protein: 5g

Peanut Butter Milkshake with Caramel

SERVES 1

1 cup coconut milk

7 ice cubes

2 tbsp. peanut butter

2 tbsp. sugar-free salted caramel syrup

1 tbsp. MCT oil

¼ tsp. xanthan gum

Peanut and caramel flavors combine deliciously in this rich, chilled dessert.

1. Add all the ingredients together in a blender, and blend until smooth. Enjoy!

NUTRITIONAL INFO PER SERVING

Calories: 365

Fat: 35g

Net Carbs: 5g

Protein: 8g

Mocha Ice Cream

SERVES 2

1 cup coconut milk

¼ cup heavy cream

2 tbsp. erythritol

16 drops liquid stevia

2 tbsp. cocoa powder

1 tbsp. instant coffee

¼ tsp. xanthan gum

Don't be fooled into thinking that you can't eat ice cream on a keto diet! Of course you can!

1. Add all the ingredients (except the xanthan gum) into an immersion blender. Blend.

2. Add xanthan gum while blending. Keep blending until the mixtures slightly thickens.

3. Put in the ice cream machine and follow the manufacturer's instructions.

NUTRITIONAL INFO PER SERVING

Calories: 146

Fat: 17g

Net Carbs: 1.7g

Protein: 2g

Chocolate Filled Peanut Butter Cookies

SERVES 20

2½ cups almond flour

½ cup peanut butter

¼ cup coconut oil

¼ cup erythritol

3 tbsp. maple syrup

1 tbsp. vanilla extract

1 ½ tsp. baking powder

½ tsp. salt

2-3 dark chocolate bars

Turn this classic recipe into a delectable keto dessert. These bites are high in fat and satisfaction!

1. Whisk the wet ingredients together.

2. Separately, mix the dry ingredients. Sift them into the wet ingredients and mix. Refrigerate for 20-30 minutes approximately.

3. Break the dark chocolate bars into small squares.

4. Form small balls of dough and press flat. Add 1 or 2 pieces of chocolate between and seal together into a ball.

5. Place on a parchment-paper-lined cookie sheet and bake at 350°F for about 15 minutes.

NUTRITIONAL INFO PER SERVING

Calories: 150

Fat: 14g

Net Carbs: 2.7g

Protein: 4.5g

Maple Nut Muffins

Serves 10

1 cup almond flour

½ cup flaxseed

¾ cup pecan (halves)

½ cup coconut oil

2 eggs

¼ cup erythritol

2 tsp. maple extract

1 tsp. vanilla extract

½ tsp. baking soda

½ tsp. apple cider vinegar

¼ tsp. liquid stevia

A great treat combining maple and pecan, and chock-full of fiber!

1. In a food processor, chop the pecans. Take ⅓ and set aside.
2. Combine all the wet ingredients in a bowl.
3. Mix the dry ingredients, and add the rest of the pecans. Add the wet ingredients and mix well.
4. In a cupcake tray, distribute the batter to make 10 muffins.
5. Over the top, sprinkle the ⅓ chopped pecans.
6. Bake at 325°F for 25-30 minutes.

Nutritional Info per Serving

Calories: 210

Fat: 20g

Net Carbs: 1.6g

Protein: 5g

Keto Bombs

Serves 2

2 tbsp. peanut butter

1 tbsp. heavy cream

1 tbsp. coconut oil

1 tsp. cocoa powder

¼ tsp. allspice

Liquid sucralose

Combine chocolate and peanut butter, and give yourself a well-deserved treat in double quick time!

1. Into a cup or mold, put the peanut butter, add the coconut oil, heavy cream, cocoa powder and allspice. Mix well.
2. Freeze for two hours and remove.

Nutritional Info per Serving

Calories: 385

Fat: 40g

Net Carbs: 8g

Protein: 8g

Easy Keto Brownie

SERVES 1

2 eggs

1 tbsp. granulated sweetener

1 scoop protein powder

1 tbsp. heavy cream

Just 3 minutes and you can have this yummy chocolaty dessert in your face!

1. In a mug, add the eggs, heavy cream, granulated sweetener and protein powder. Mix well.

2. Microwave for 1 minute.

NUTRITIONAL INFO PER SERVING

Calories: 310

Fat: 15g

Net Carbs: 5g

Protein: 35g

Keto Peanut Butter Ice Cream

SERVES 2

1 cup cottage cheese

2 tbsp. protein powder

2 tbsp. peanut butter

2 tbsp. heavy cream

6 drops liquid sweetener

Craving ice cream? Try this easy peanut butter variation loaded with protein and fats.

1. Put the cottage cheese, sweetener, heavy cream, and peanut butter into a food processor. Blend until the curds have been chopped up and the mixture is smooth.

2. Add protein powder, and blend again.

3. Freeze for 40 minutes.

NUTRITIONAL INFO PER SERVING

Calories: 170

Fat: 10g

Net Carbs: 2g

Protein: 15g

Low-Carb Cookies

Serves 18

2½ cups blanched almond flour

¼ cup shelled and chopped walnuts

½ cup unsalted butter

2 eggs

½ cup powdered erythritol

½ cup dark chocolate chips

Salt

½ tsp. baking soda

1 tbsp. vanilla extract

A classic turned into this healthy option for you and the kids. Make them as a family activity!

1. In a bowl, combine almond flour, salt, baking soda and erythritol.

2. Separately, mix melted butter and vanilla, chocolate chips, eggs and walnuts. Combine with the dry mixture until you have dough.

3. Make cookies with 1 scoop of the dough per cookie and place them onto a cookie sheet. 4. Bake for 8-10 at 350°F. Cool for 10 minutes.

Nutritional Info per Serving

Calories: 172

Fat: 15g

Net Carbs: 3g

Protein: 0g

Microwave Brownie

Serves 1

1 tbsp. creamy almond butter

1 tbsp. beaten egg white

1 tsp. unsweetened cocoa powder

⅛ tsp. vanilla extract

3 drops liquid sucralose or stevia

Baking soda

Salt

Almonds or pecans, orange or lemon extract (optional)

For busy people who crave a brownie dessert, this recipe will become a go-to for when you're short on time.

1. Beat egg whites in a bowl until they are frothy.

2. In a microwave-safe cup, mix the egg white mixture with the rest of the ingredients.

3. Microwave for 40 seconds and remove.

Nutritional Info per Serving

Calories: 105

Fat: 9g

Net Carbs: 3g

Protein: 0g

Dark Chocolate Brownie

Serves 16

6 tbsp. cream cheese

3 eggs

3 tbsp. coconut oil

2 tbsp. heaped cocoa powder

¼ cup almond flour

¼ cup coconut flour

¼ tbsp. baking soda

9 packets truvia

½ cup almond milk

1 tsp. vanilla extract

Salt

These brownies are legendary. They are great source of healthy fats, and really help you out when you are craving something sweet.

1. In a bowl, combine the cheese, eggs, coconut oil, almond milk and vanilla extract.

2. In another bowl, mix the dry ingredients: cocoa powder, almond flour, coconut flour, baking soda, truvia and a bit of salt. When done, incorporate the wet ingredients and mix well.

3. Pour the batter into a cake pan. Cook for 30 minutes at 375°F. Let them cool for a few minutes.

Nutritional Info per Serving

Calories: 76

Fat: 8g

Net Carbs: 4g

Protein: 3g

Chocolate Cookies

Serves 16

7 tbsp. butter

2 cups almond flour

¾ cup granulated sweetener

2 oz. dark chocolate

2 eggs

1 tbsp. orange zest

1 tbsp. orange juice

1 tsp. orange extract

1 tsp. vanilla extract

¾ tsp. baking powder

½ tsp. baking soda

½ tsp. salt

Is it obvious we love cookies? With almost 15g carbs and 20g protein per serving, it's easy to see why.

1. Mix the almond flour, baking soda, baking powder, salt, and granulated sweetener.

2. Melt the butter in a microwave-safe bowl and then mix it with the orange juice, orange zest, orange extract and vanilla extract.

3. Combine both mixtures and add the broken-up chocolate and eggs. Make sure they are well mixed.

4. Place the dough oven a baking sheet on a cookie sheet, forming rectangles and cut it into 16.

5. Bake at 350°F for about 20-25 minutes.

Nutritional Info per Serving

Calories: 155

Fat: 14g

Net Carbs: 10g

Protein: 17g

Low Carb Shortbread

Serves 24

2 cups almond flour

½ tsp. baking soda

½ tsp. baking powder

⅓ cup granulated sweetener

6 tbsp. butter

1 tsp. vanilla extract

1 tbsp. lemon zest, grated

4 tsp. lemon juice

2 tsp. rosemary, dried or fresh

The lemon and rosemary in this low carb shortbread make a world of difference. Make a batch and share them out with friends and family.

1. In a bowl, combine almond flour, baking powder, baking soda and sweetener.

2. Melt the butter in a microwave, and add the vanilla extract, lemon zest, lemon juice and rosemary. Incorporate the dried mixture stirring slowly. When done, wrap the dough in a plastic wrap and place in the freezer for 30 minutes.

3. Remove the dough from the freezer, and cut it into 12 pieces.

4. Bake for 15 minutes at 350°F on a greased cookie sheet with salted butter. When done, let cool for 10 minutes.

Nutritional Info per Serving

Calories: 80

Fat: 7g

Net Carbs: 1g

Protein: 2g

Keto White Chocolate Bark

Serves 12

2 oz. cocoa butter

⅓ cup low-carb sweetener

1 tsp. vanilla powder

½ tsp. hemp seed powder

1 tsp. toasted pumpkin seeds

Salt

This awesome option is made with cocoa butter, which will change your perspective on chocolate altogether.

1. Chop the cocoa butter into fine pieces.

2. Prepare a double boiler. Put the water in the outer pot and place the cocoa butter in the inner pot. Melt over a medium heat.

3. Mix the remaining ingredients.

4. Grease a small bowl with coconut oil. When the cocoa butter is melted, mix with the rest of the ingredients and pour into the greased bowl.

5. Let the mixture cool, then remove from the bowl and break into 12 pieces.

Nutritional Info per Serving

Calories: 40

Fat: 2 grams

Net Carbs: 0g

Protein: 0g

Low Carb Chocolate

SERVES 24

1 cup expeller-pressed coconut oil

1 cup cocoa powder

⅔ cup granulated sweetener

This basic recipe goes well with all your treats. Combine with keto cupcakes and cookies, and consider yourself an expert chef!

1. In a double boiler over a medium heat, melt the coconut oil.

2. Combine the cocoa powder and sweetener. Add the melted oil and mix well.

3. Let it cool.

NUTRITIONAL INFO PER SERVING

Calories: 100

Fat: 9g

Net Carbs: 1g

Protein: 0.8g

Avocado Smoothie

Serves 1

3 oz. unsweetened almond milk

3 oz. heavy whipping cream

6 drops sweetener

1 avocado

7 ice cubes

A simple, delicious smoothie that doesn't need any prep; simply blend and go!

1. In a blender, add the almond milk, the avocado, ice and blend them until smooth.

Nutritional Info per Serving

Calories: 588

Fat: 60g

Net Carbs: 20g

Protein: 5g

Vodka Whipped Cream

SERVES 10

200 ml. heavy cream

¼ tsp. vanilla

¼ tsp. liquid sucralose

50 ml. vanilla vodka

Vodka whipped cream is all the rage, and can be expensive. But you can make your own for a lot less!

1. Whip the cream until it begins to form soft peaks. Add the sucralose and part of the vodka, and continue whipping.

2. When the peaks become stiff, add the remaining vodka and whip until the desired consistency is achieved.

NUTRITIONAL INFO PER SERVING

Calories: 230

Fat: 100g

Net Carbs: 0g

Protein: 0g

Keto Macaroons

Serves 1

4 egg whites

1 tsp. vanilla

1 cup artificial sweetener

4½ tsp. water

½ cup unsweetened coconut

Delicious coconut flavored macaroons that are as close to the original as you can get.

1. Mix the white eggs with the liquid ingredients. Add the coconut and mix. Blend with an immersion blender to achieve a nicer consistency.

2. Place the batter on a greased pie pan and bake for 15 minutes at 325°F.

Nutritional Info per Serving

Calories: 90

Fat: 10g

Net Carbs: 4g

Protein: 2g

Low Carb Cheesecake

SERVES 8

The Crust

¾ cup pecans, crushed

¾ cup almond flour

4 tbsp. butter

2 tbsp. granulated sweetener

The Filling

1½ lbs cream cheese

4 eggs

½ tbsp. liquid vanilla

½ tbsp. lemon juice

1 cup granulated sweetener

¼ cup sour cream

9 strawberries

A classic dessert turned keto. Prepare it and share the good news with your keto friends.

1. In a saucepan, melt the butter and add crushed pecans, sweetener and almond flour. Mix for few minutes until they are combined.

2. Grease a spring-form pan and spread the crust in the bottom, packing it down.

3. Make the filling by combining all the ingredients at room temperature, mixing well until smooth.

4. Put sliced strawberries on the top of the crust, add the filling and then another layer of sliced strawberries.

5. Bake for 60-90 minutes at 250°F. Let it cool and place in the fridge until ready to serve.

NUTRITIONAL INFO PER SERVING

Calories: 540

Fat: 50g

Net Carbs: 10g

Protein: 15g

FREE BONUS GUIDE:

Top 10 Keto Diet Mistakes

We hope you enjoy making your way through the delicious meals contained in this cookbook, and want to offer you a little something extra to ensure you stay safe and maximize your results.

With our free bonus guide you will learn the top 10 mistakes people make when cooking keto, and discover exactly how to avoid them for yourself. Curious? Use the link below to see it now!

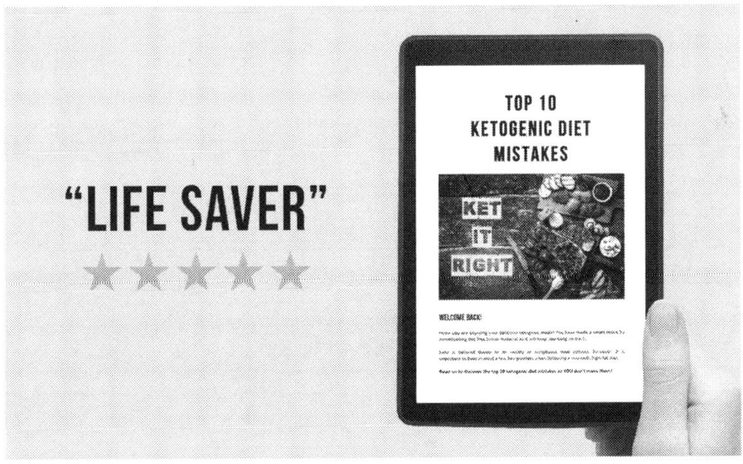

Visit http://geni.us/ketomistakes to get your copy now!

Like This Book?

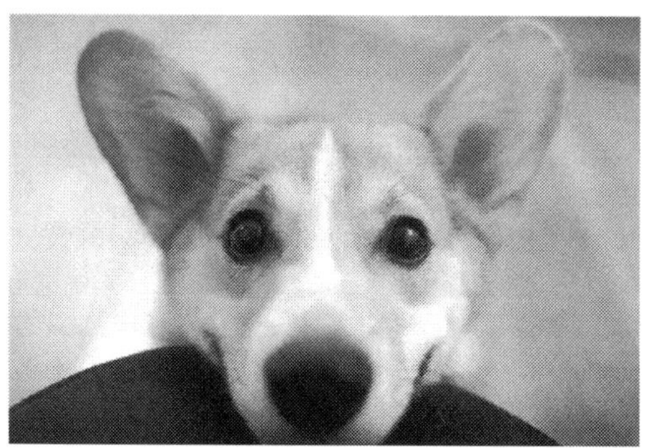

This is Buster, and he'd really love to know what you thought!

If you got value from this book, or the free bonus guide, it would be amazing if you could visit your Amazon order history to leave a quick review. You can even upload a picture of your favorite recipe! Oh, and don't forget to share the love with a friend!

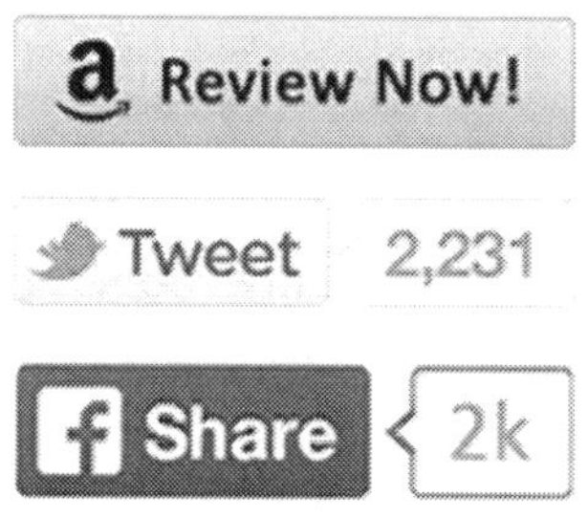

77532363R00081

Made in the USA
Lexington, KY
28 December 2017